1

What Is KO?

Takuya Futaesaku

&

Fightology World Team

DEDICATION

This book is dedicated to
PRINCE & JOHN BLACKWELL

"For all of us, life is death without adventure, and adventure only
comes to those who are willing to be daring and take chances."
Prince 1958-4ever

ACKNOWLEDGMENTS

I would love to thank my family. Hiroko, Sheila, Nate, Mam, Dad,
and Toru. All of my friends in fighting world, thank you so much for
standing on my corner, not only in good times but in bad times. I
would love to show my love to my special friends in music world.
You all are my heroes and great inspiration. Arigato Gozaimasu.
Dr. F

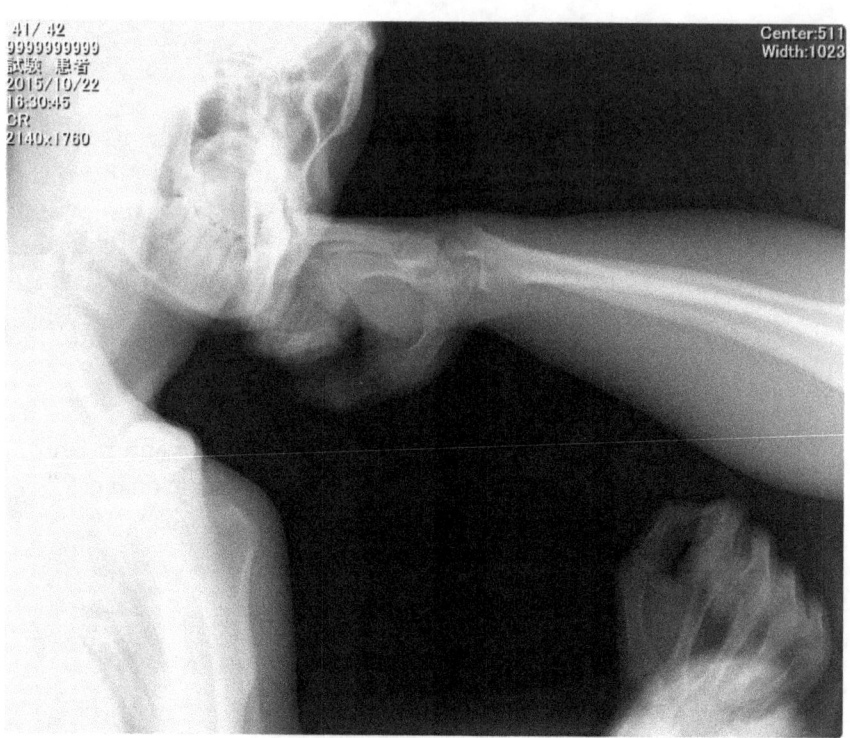

FIGHTOLOGY WORLD TEAM

HIROSHI KATSUI/MAURICIO CARRANZA/
FABIO ROSCH/MOISÉS FALLAS WAHRMANN/
JUAN MA Z PIEDRA/DAVID ORSINI/
DAN NAKAMURA/HON KUEN MA/
MASASHI   SAITO/HIDEO KATO/
JUAN CARLOS AUGE ROS/JASON LAM/
DANIEL PEREZ/JASON DROGUETT/
ANGUS WONG/CHI KIN FUNG/GAVIN SZETO

CONTENTS

1:What Is KO? -Brain-

2:What Is KO? -Body-

3:What Is KO? -Low Kick-

4:What Is KO? -KO sense-

1:WHAT IS KO?
-BRAIN-

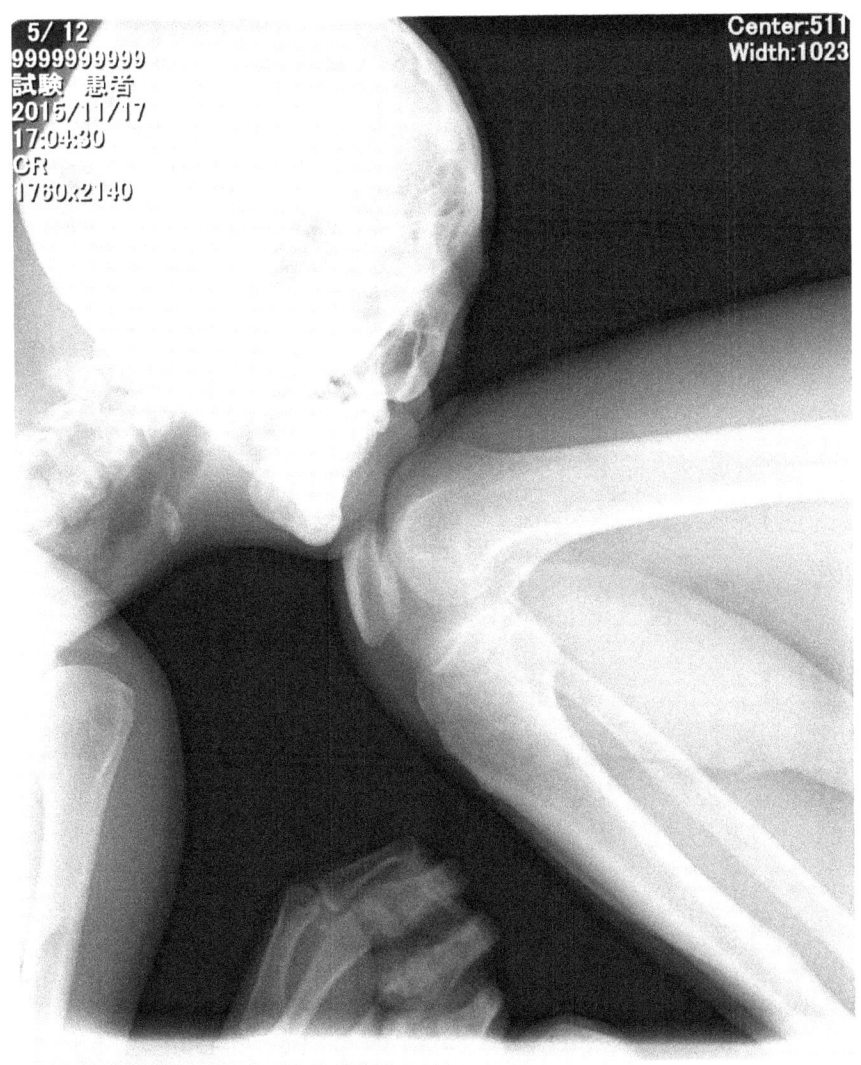

1-1 【KO in facial attack】

A reversal KO by a punch of a boxing fighter, win by ippon with a brilliant high kick of a Karateka, an elbow strike when crossing each other by Muaythai warrior, a spectacular fainting KO by a mixed martial artist's pound .... After a momentary silence, the venue is wrapped in a cheer that makes the ear hurt! Everyone who wants to train fighting sports and martial arts, must dream of a knockout win. It is not a subtle victory in judgment, I want to win clearly with KO, I want to prove my strength, there are many people who sweat every day with such feelings! However, the game is a serious game. Far from KO, the real world is that even a victory by decision is not an easy thing. No matter how much the fans shout "Defeat! Defeat!", seeing from the outside and actually standing in front of the opponent is totally different thing.

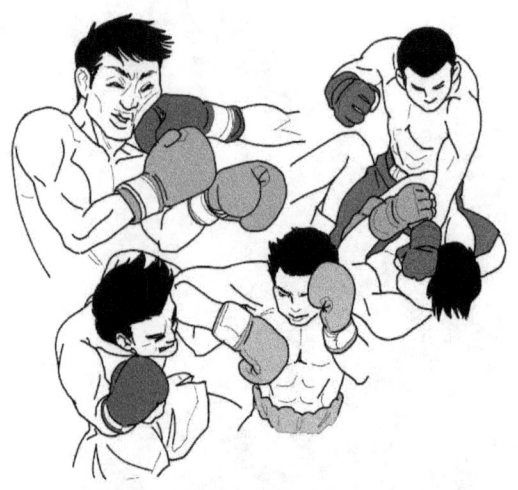

Technique that has polished with sandbags, mitts, sparring thousands of times or even tens of thousands of times by tolerating what you like such as play and alcohol. Clean hit on your opponent's face in the game! Even though I feel a certain response ... the opponent is still standing there without falling down.

"Why?"
"Is my power insufficient? "
"The timing is bad?"
" Am I slow? "
"Is my opponent too tough?"
"Was my condition bad?"
"Don't I have the talent on martial arts?"
"Is martial art not for me?"

Please wait a moment, let's think about how "KO" will happen in a system before deciding to think so. Why will we fall from being attacked above the neck? That is because the brain shakes rapidly due to external force, concussion occurs where the nerve function stops]. Knockout by attacking on the face is a technique to cause the opponent to concussion. Although the mechanism by which concussion occurs is not fully elucidated. It is considered, when a radical physical stimulus is added to the brain, the brain judges that "if it is more active there is a risk of life" in order to protect the brain itself and the body, it stops consciousness, senses and movements.

1-2 【Rotation of head and structure of cervical vertebra】

Analyzing KO scenes in fighting sports and martial arts with slow motion movies, you could observe the head rotates in most cases. So what kind of secret is hidden in the technique of shaking the brain by rotating the head rapidly? Let's explore in detail the structure where the head rotates. The head is on the neck. There are seven bones in the neck which is called cervical vertebrae, for mammals. Even a strong fighter like monster has seven. There is no such case like there are 8 for a fighter whose character is unique and strange.The top of the cervical vertebra is called the 1st cervical vertebra, its alias is , atlas, shaped like a ring. The skull is on the atlas, and since both are stuck together in the tissue, the skull + atlas moves almost in unison. And the second cervical vertebra is characterized by a protrusion that protrudes towards the head, it is called the axial vertebra or axis. The atlas rests on the dens which is the shaft part of this shaft, forming a joint called atlanto-axial joint. With the dens as the central axis, the atlas rotates with the circle. In the movement of the cervical vertebra, there are a head tilting forward (flexing), tilting the head to the back (extension), tilting the head left and right (side bending), turning left and right (rotation), especially the annular joint moves mainly.

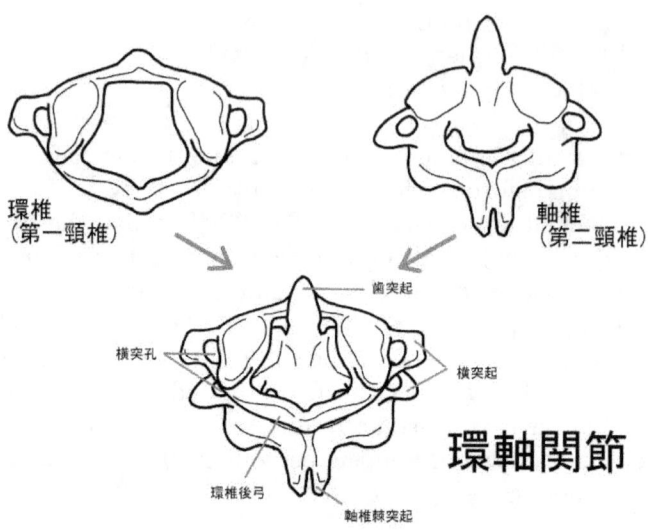

環椎 : atlas
軸椎 : axis
環軸関節 : atlanto-axial joint

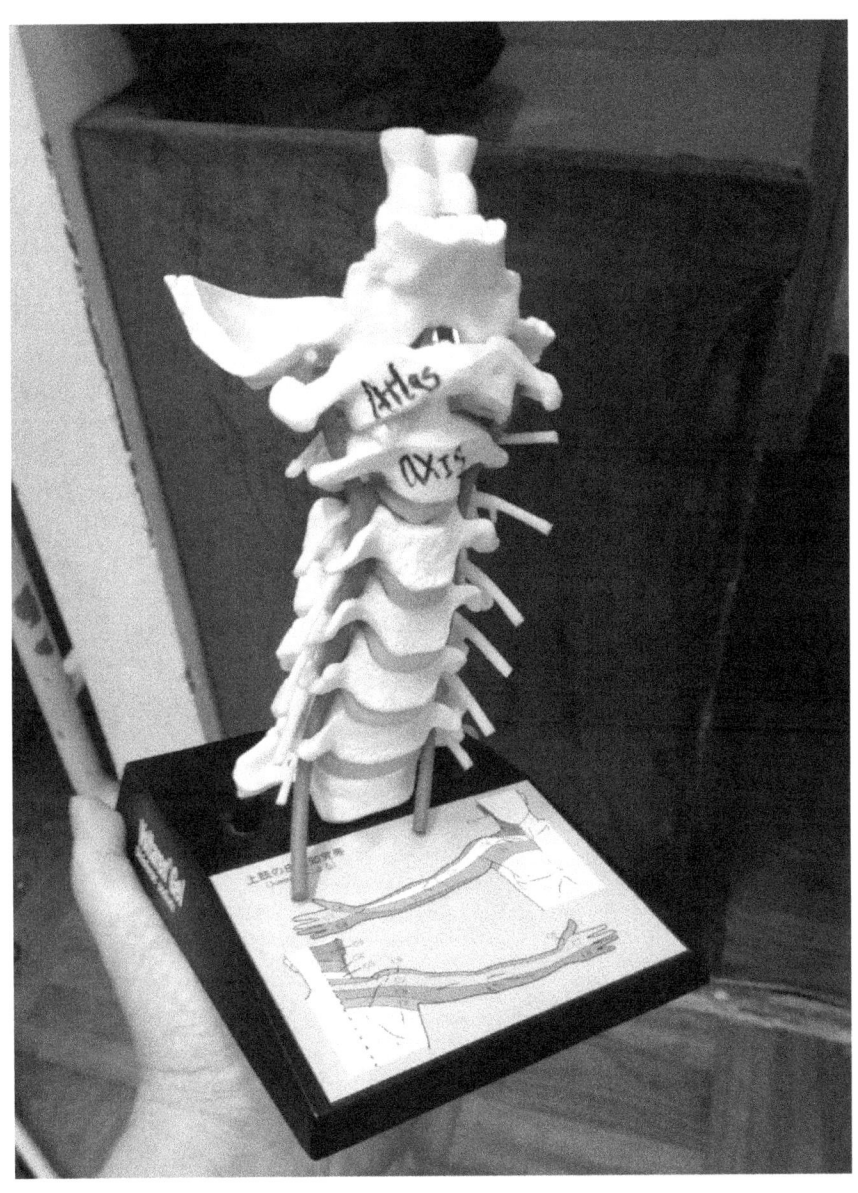

1-3 【Condition of KO Part 1 ~ Course ~】

One of the reasons why punches and kicks do not collapse even if they hit the opponent's face, chin, temple, etc. has a problem of the striking course. In order to shake the brain, we must move the annulus joint dynamically with external force. For striking course that can not defeat the opponent, is that external forces due to punches and kicks tend to head toward the center of the atlanto-axial joint. In this course, since it is difficult to apply force in the direction of rotation, it is difficult to shake the head even with a strong blow. Since it strikes against the center of atlanto-axial joint, the reaction of the blow is great, the response of the blows and the kicks is steady. If you do not understand the principle, you tend to think that you are "Hitting firmly but not knocking him down, so how about a course of blows that can knockdown? The knocking down strike will move away from the center of the atlanto-axial joint after hitting. Kicking the soccer ball which is held still, you'd rather kick deviating from the center than kicking the center. With this principle, in order to rotate the head, a course that makes force not going to the center of the joint is likely to be connected to KO. The reason why you don't feel reaction against your fist or foot when you KO the opponent by striking the opponent's head is because the striking goes through the course of KO.

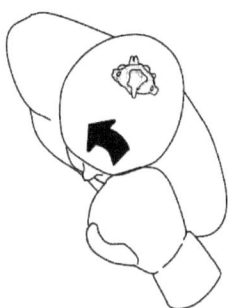 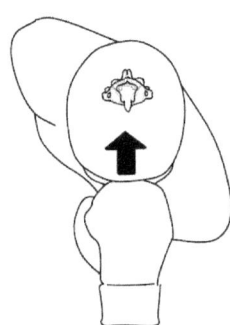

Make a partner and the fighter slowly places his fists and feet on his partner's face, looking for a course of KO with slow motion while giving due consideration to avoid injury. Please try various kinds of punches and kicks while changing hit points such as chin, cheekbones, temple. In the world of fighting sports, it is sometimes adjective to the types of fighters, such as "His chin is weak" or "Jaw of glass". For players whose distance from the atlanto-axial joint to the lower jaw is long, the head is easy to rotate by the length of the diameter. Conversely round faced fighters and short necked fighters are harder to rotate than players who are not so, it is said that it is difficult for the head to rotate even if you target the chin.

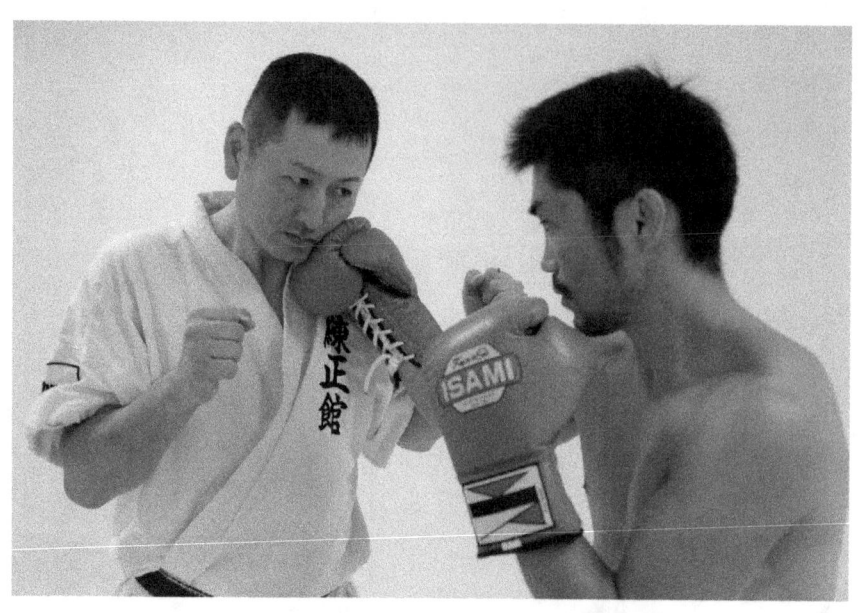

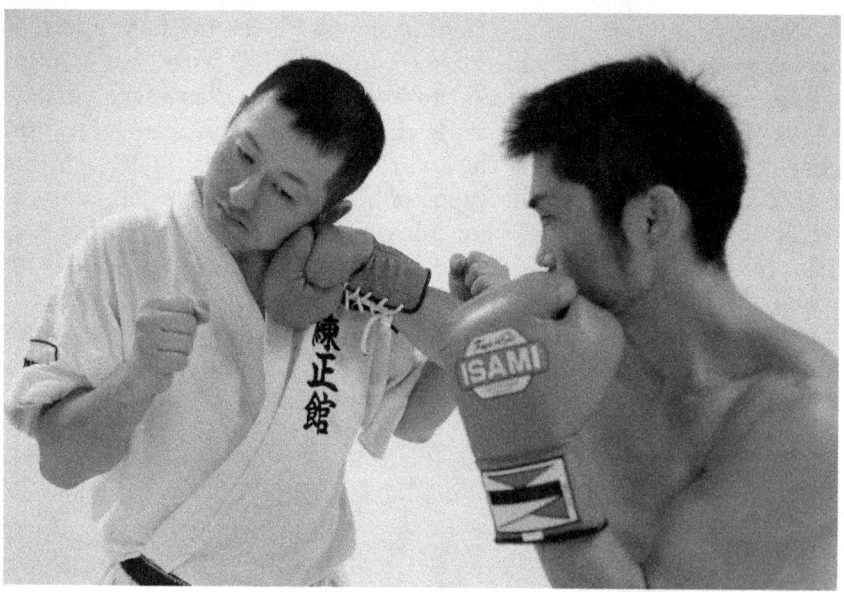

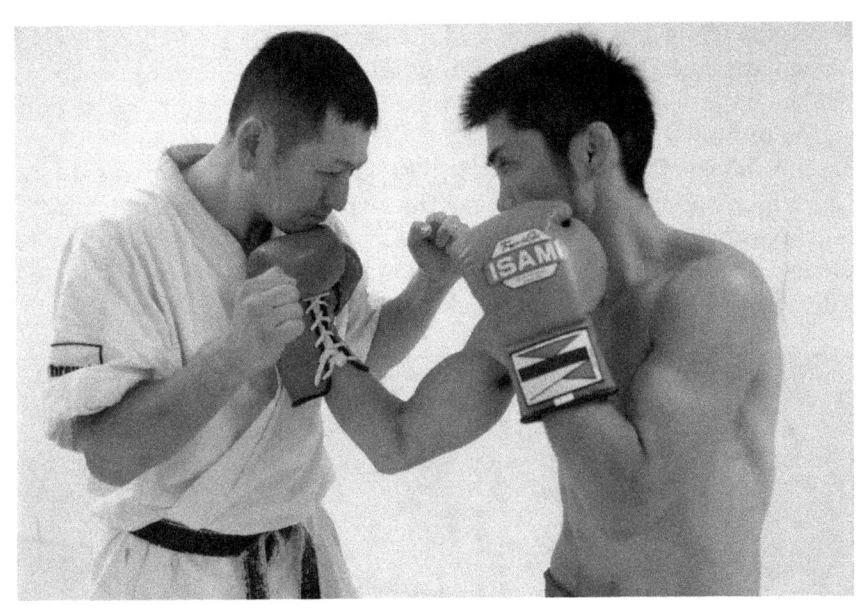

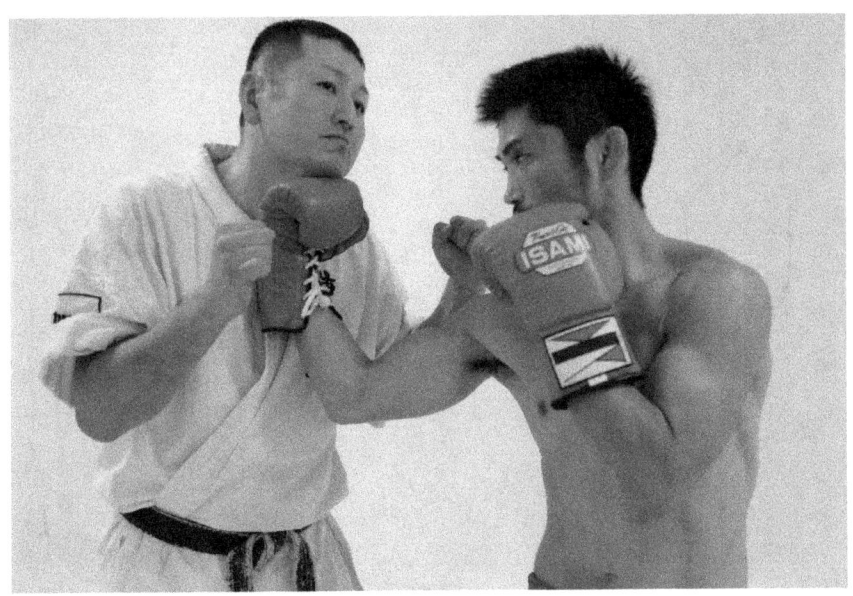

In the Society of Fighting Medicine, we took the X-ray of cervical vertebrae and head, and measured
(A) the distance from the atlanto-axial joint to the lower jaw tip
(B) the distance from the atlanto-axial joint to the temporal region, as temple
on the flat surface. As a result, (A) was 13.20 cm, (B) was 14.59 cm, which the result was larger than the other parts. (Actually it is three dimensional and there are individual differences, so please regard it as a reference value only.) It resulted to be inferred the reason for aiming chin and temple, from X-ray.

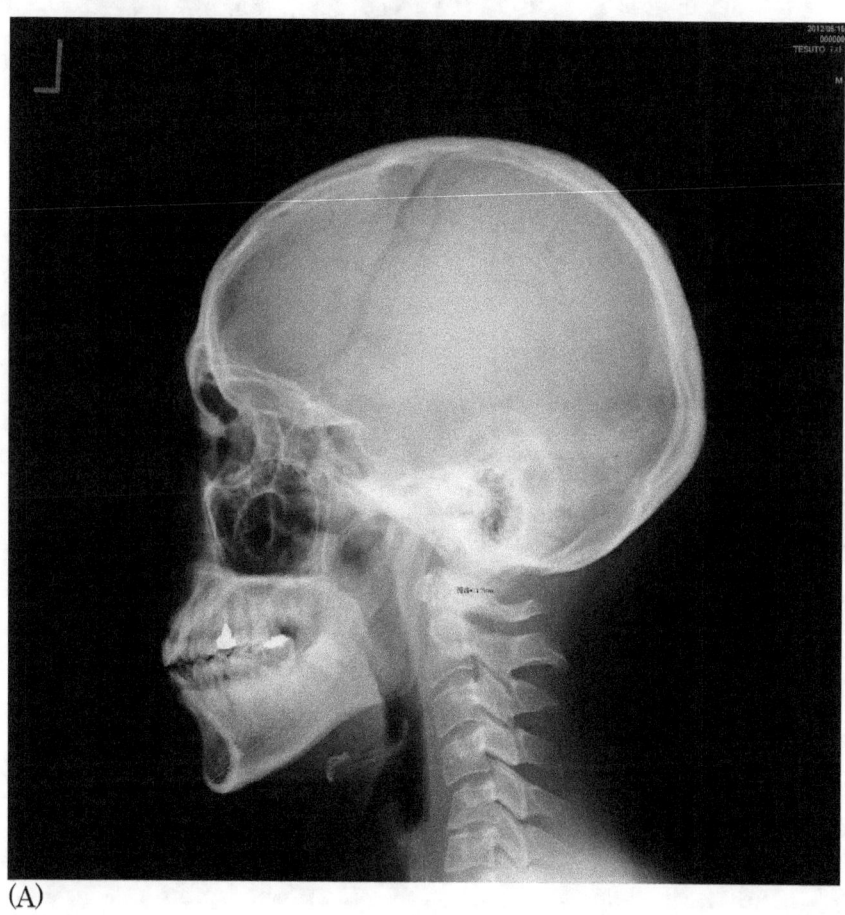

(A)

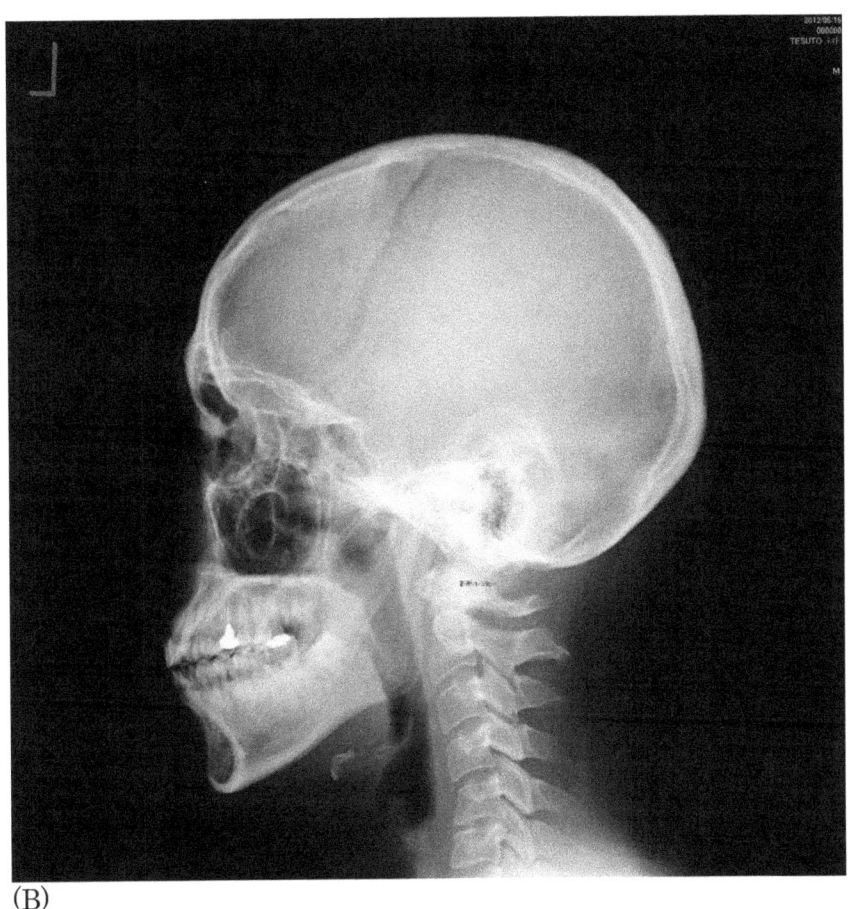

(B)

One boxing world champion has changes the aiming point by the type such as the shape of the partner's face, the muscles mass, the direction of the neck, and so on. As expected it is a world champion class, databases to knock down are accumulated in the brain and body! Look for the parts you should hit your punch and kick, and the courses that turns the head and the direction of the force with consciousness in the condition of the trusted relationship with your partner.

1-4 【Condition of KO Part 2 ~ Speed ~】

To shake the brain, you have to make the head 'rapidly rotate'. For that purpose, let's control the speed so that it will be the fastest speed from the moment you hit it until the rotation takes place. If you are doing sandbags and mitts at the practice stage all the time, your consciousness to control this speed may be weaken. In the case of a bag or mitt, the motion stops for a moment immediately after hitting the punch or kick. To stop will mean "the speed will be zero." As a result, when the most speed is required, the brain and the body will learn to "stop when the attacks hit". It is a really wasteful story that there are athletes piling punches that can not KO, with a mistake in choosing a practicing method while still having the speed that can make a KO. As a way to train the KO speed, here we will introduce what we can apply from among methods actually being done by the champion class fighters.

1. Towel kick, towel punch

Practice punching and kicking through the towel which only is fixed at the top edge. Since the reaction from the moment you hit is small, you can trim your skills at maximum speed. The faster the speed, the sharp explosion sounds, so you can evaluate the degree of completion of the skill by "sound". In my team, we do the warming up with towel for the kicks which goes through, with mitt for the pulling back kicks before the game. For the warming up of the world champion of kickboxing, once the towel was torn up by a single high kick.

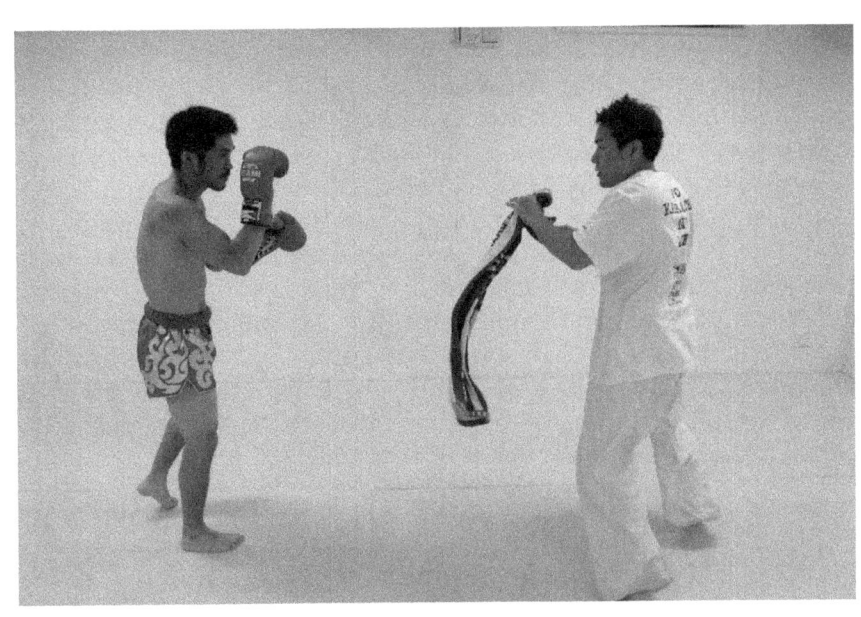

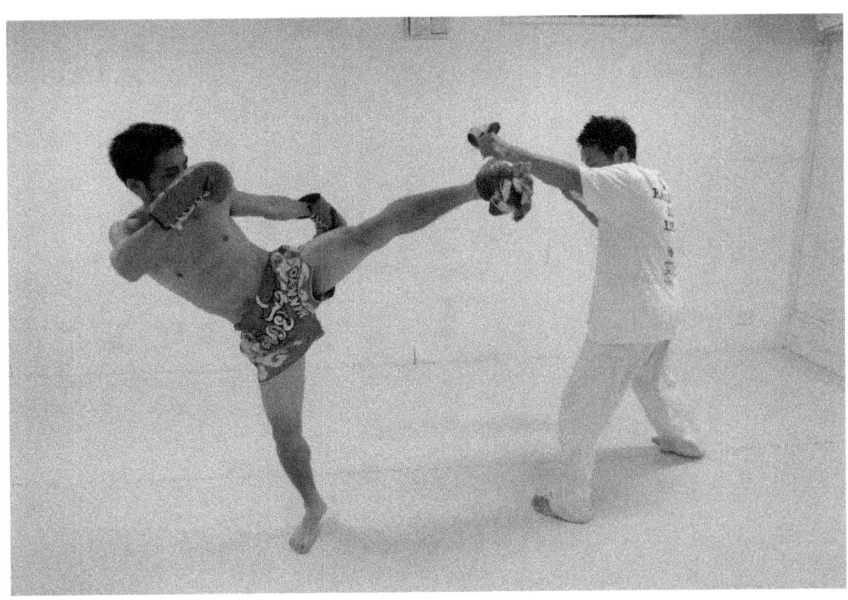

23

2. Momentum mitt

This is a practice to shorten the contact time of the technique. Do not hold the mit tightly, and receive with the relaxed shoulder joint and the elbow joint and give each joint a little room for its movement. In order to rotate the head rapidly, it is necessary to minimize the time when gloves, fists, and kicking legs are hit. For example, in the case of a straight punch, the mitt goes back to the back as it follows, even if there is a speed of the punch, the time it touches is long, becoming a pushing punch and it will become difficult to knockdown the opponent. At the moment when you hit, try practicing mitt to change the course into "cut" like strike at the moment of impact. It is also effective to draw a mark on the mitt and draw an arrow in the direction to cut. Please practice with care so that the blow will not stay at the place you hit.

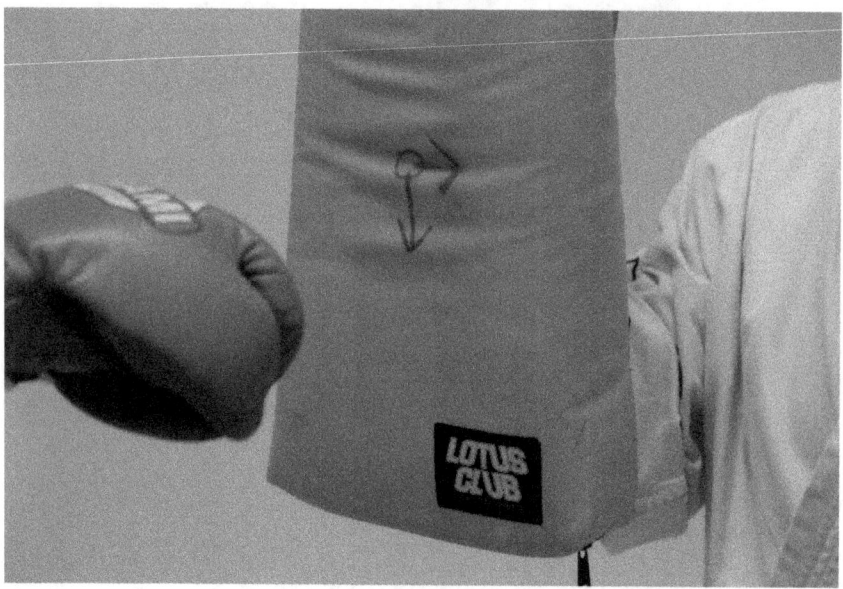

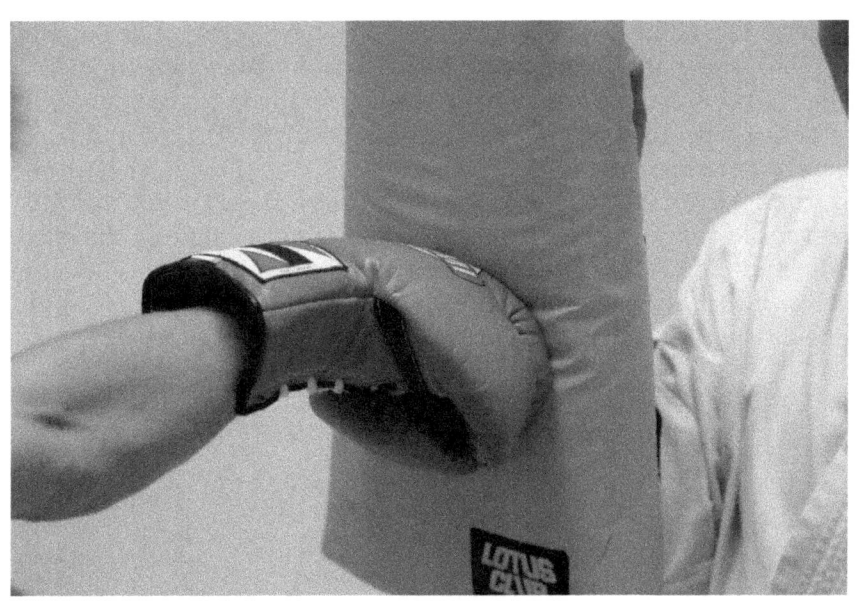

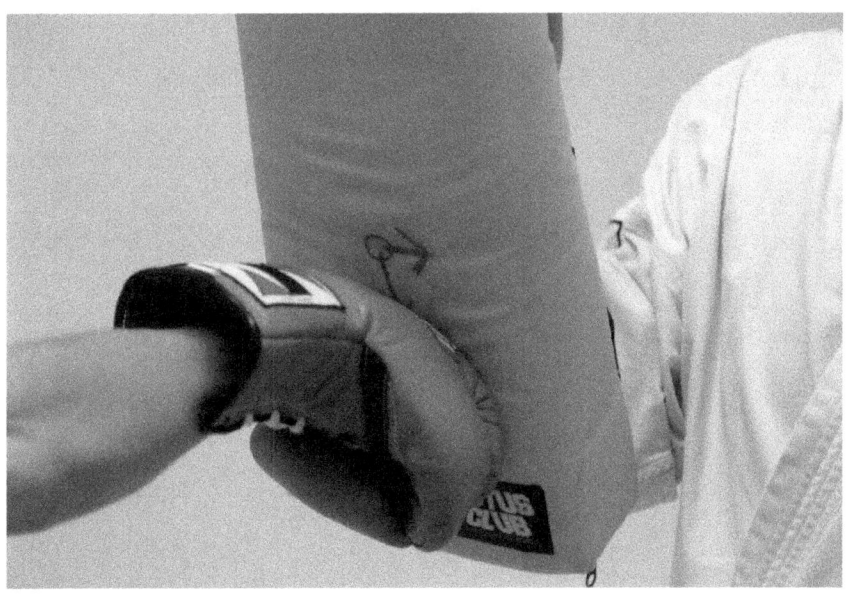

3, speed tube

Practice techniques using a tube. The partner applies tension, so that the maximum speed comes out at the moment of hit. Normally, we strike against the tension of the tube, but that way is only a very useful way to improve muscular strength and learn how to use the body, but the drawback is that the longer the tube is, the load gets bigger and the speed drops. In order to solve this, leave it to the tension of the tube, and by partner pulling the edge, adjust to the maximum speed strike will be realized when the strike hits. As the brain and body memorize more speed than usual, you can expect an improvement in speed.

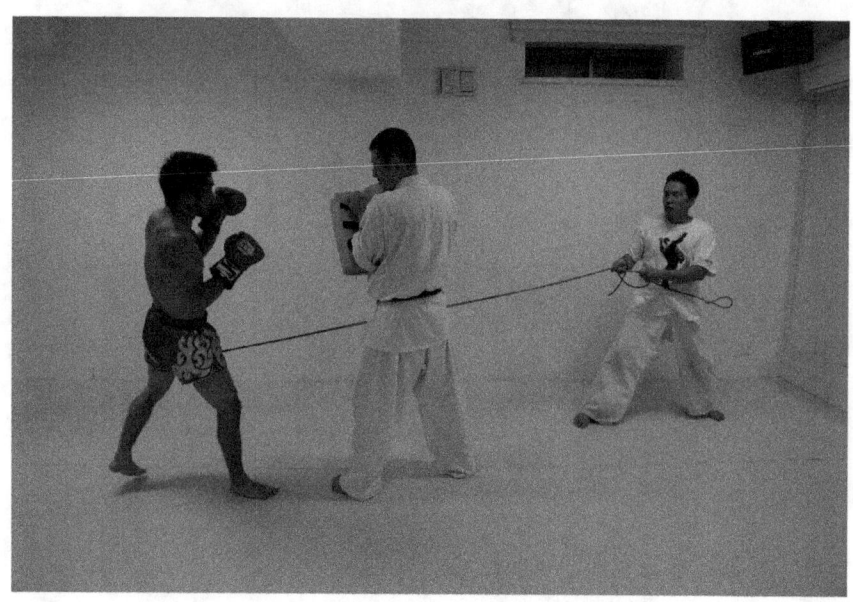

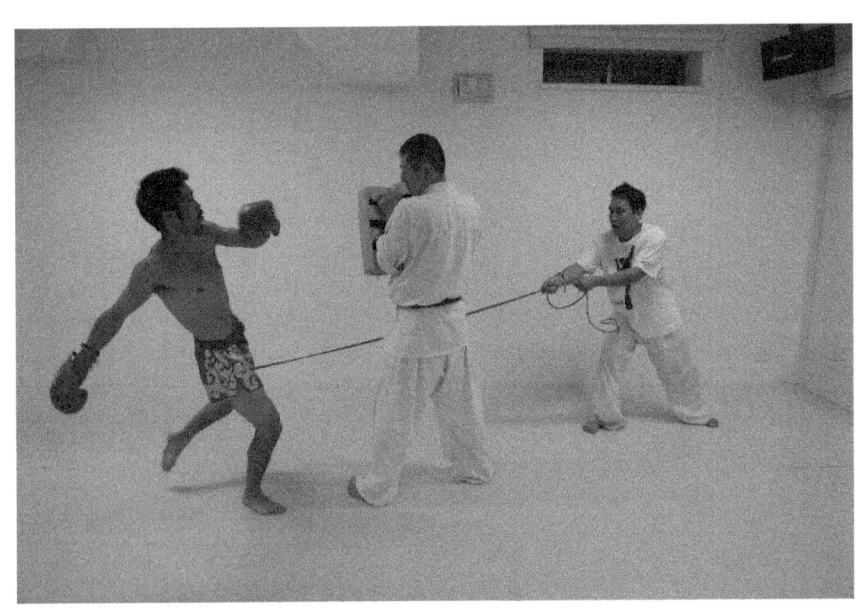

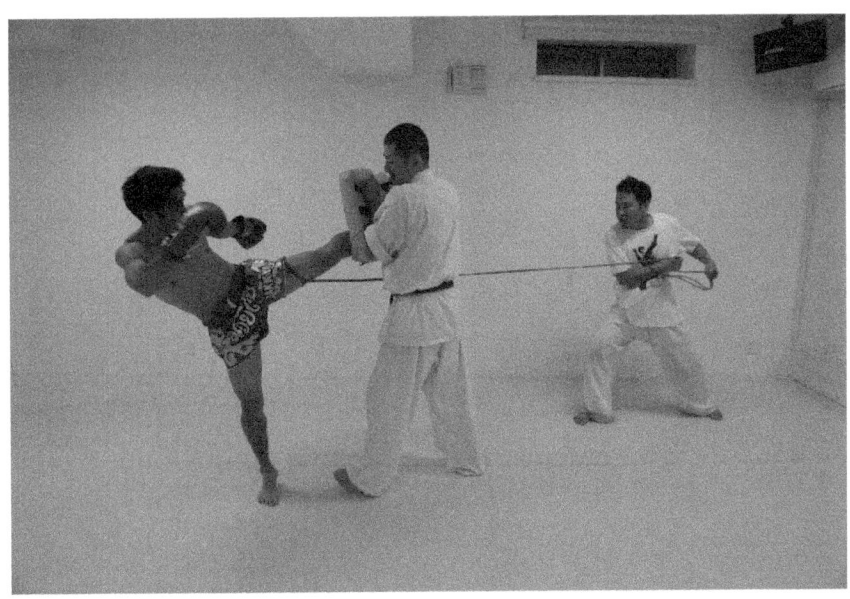

27

The important thing with KO is speed control. Take the speed of the moment of hit as important as to reach the maximum speed so that your fists or gloves disappear, or your legs disappear if that is kicks. Since fighting sports and martial arts competitions are interpersonal competitions, it is also effective to input the speed to your opponent. You may show the opponent a slow blow several times and make it fast sometimes. Also, keep moving fast and combine slow blows. When it comes to a top fighter, at the start up, punching and kicking slowly, pulling out slow reactions, then rapidly accelerating. Even in one technique, they will interweave control of speed. Speed is important to KO, but there are actually fighters who can KO even if the speed is not so fast. So, even if the movement is late, you do not have to give up KO. I'd like you to raise your awareness of "controlling" the speed while seeking the fastest among them.

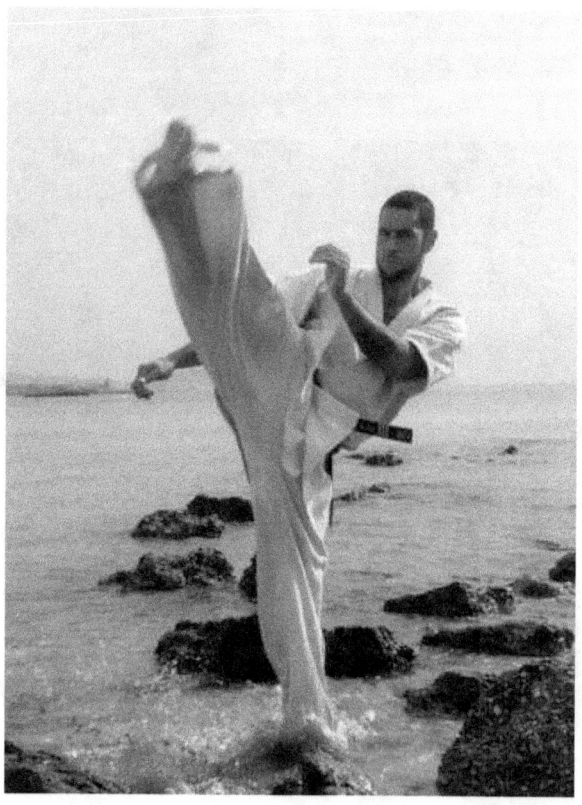

1-5【Condition of KO Part 3 ~ Surprise ~】

The first-class fighter is first-rate not to mention knock out "technique" is first class, but "method" to ensure that the technique is hit is also top notch. By analyzing the behavior of KO artists, you can approach the secret of that method.

"Ironman" Mike Tyson

If you ask people who the strongest boxer of the heavyweight class is, either Mike Tyson or Muhammad Ali will be named. Mike Tyson as he is only 180cm short and small body mass as a heavy weight class fighter amongst the fighters whom are like dinosaurs and easily more than 190cm tall, produces KO with overwhelming power and speed, not only for the fistiana, he is a legendary boxer that can make its name in the other fighting sports and the other sports society. 12th and 19th WBC, 34th and 42nd WBA, 4th IBF, World Heavyweight Champion. The 50 wins of 58 matches , 44 games were victories with KO, the heyday is in a state "knockout if hit". It was the time, even the people whom have no interest in fighting sports nor boxing, had paid attention, and been excited to see him how many seconds he is going to take, to knockout the opponent, in front of the TV.   It was a player who embodied one punch KO which is the real thrill of heavyweight boxing.

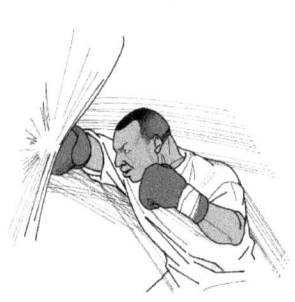

Mike Tyson has developed around the waist, girth, shoulder, chest, neck and muscle, and muscle power and speed are also super high level. He transforms the jumping force created around a tough lower body, and hip joint, convert purely into hook and upper. It is a fight style which is called Peek-A-Boo, a style that hides the face behind the gloves, approaches the opponent and jumps into the close distance. In this state I took an X-ray, the lower jaw is securely protected with both fists, and furthermore the lower edge of the lower jaw is approaching the clavicle and the risk that Tyson will be KOed even at the meeting distance, it is reducing it.

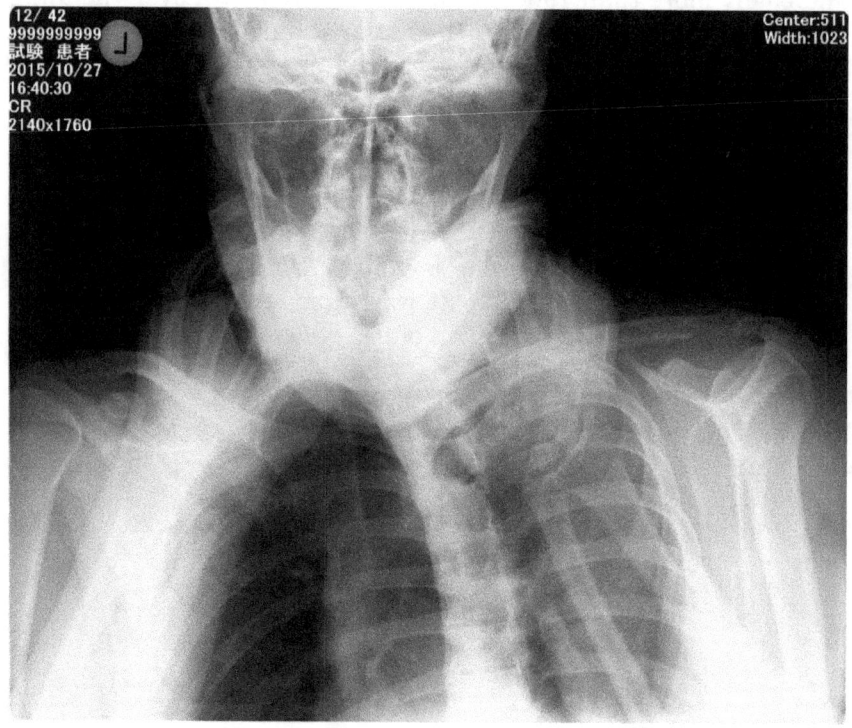

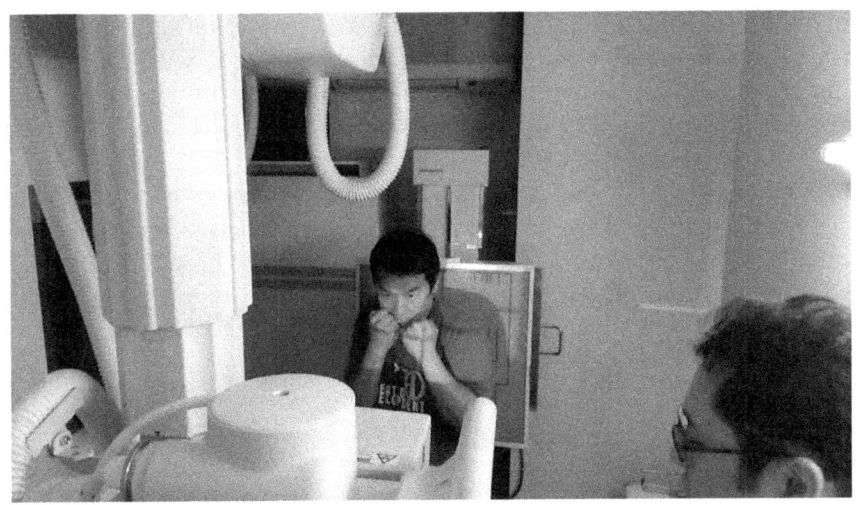

How many times we acclaim Tyson's overwhelming physical ability, it is never enough. but its "art" is also a first-class item. Tyson walks up to me straight while guarding it to the distance before the opponent's punch reaches. As far as you can see the image of Tyson, there seems to be no option to pull back basically. Most of the time he moves forward in the matches. This means that when viewed from the opponent's side, the image reflected on the retina is getting bigger and bigger. As the image grows big, humans feel psychological pressure and fear. That is the same case as if a dump truck which is going away it is not scary, but when it is chasing you, that is scary. Tyson who is pretty small in the heavyweight, in a match he comes closer and closer, so the information is inputted as a large object to the opponent. When the round starts, he walks straight up to the opponent. After referee breaks, he walks straight up to the opponent again. Giving pressure and walk to the opponent from long distance, then suddenly disappears at the meeting distance! He isn't actually an invisible man and disappear but while pivoting the hip joint, the pelvis is dropped in the direction of gravity, and furthermore the whole body is rolled while bending the torso and "drops" in the direction of gravity, so the pelvis and head height are displaced downwards by several tens of centimeters. At the next moment, Tyson delivers hooks and uppers while jumping dynamically like a frog flying off the surface of the water. To the opponent, "He give me pressure by walking straight up to me all the time from long distance, becomes small and disappears from the sight when I thought it was my distance, at the next moment, with the large image of Tyson right in front of my eyes, a punch which is accurate like no other blows toward me." I might say. That is literally Peek-A-Boo! The style just like that play, people were being knocked out whenever it hit. Overwhelming basic physical strength + the perfect tactics which give us surprise. The shocking impact that we had at Tyson's heyday, I feel these 2 elements were inside, simultaneously.

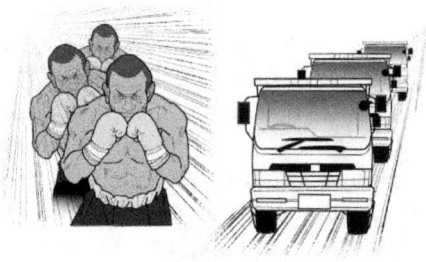

There is an anecdote, Constantine "Cus" D'Amato, a famous trainer who discovered Tyson's talent at Tyson's childhood and brought him up, charged Tyson 25kg heavy weight luggage on his shoulder to go to school at his growth period. Instead of making a small physique bigger, make it even smaller and larger and give the opponent a surprise. Constantine "Cus" D'Amato led by converting the disadvantage of being short in height into advantage as "use lower space advantageously than opponent". "Make a form which is hard to be knocked down and easy to move" "Become small and become large" "Keep giving pressure on the opponent" "Sharp up the basic physical strength and speed" "Jab is the basic technic of punches. strike with whole body" and so on. The art of the legendary ironman Mike Tyson who mass-produced KOs, it would be the strongest hint for the fighters with not gifted of his body mass or anyone who has to fight against a huge opponent.

"Devil Prince" Naseem Hamed

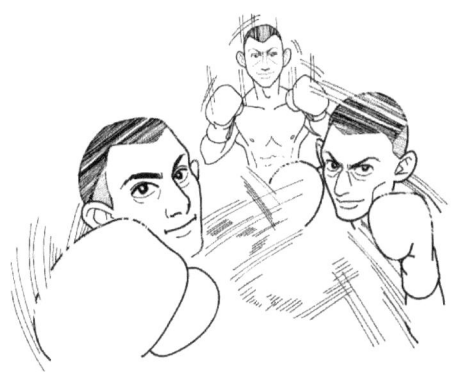

The most revolutionary fighter in boxing history that built a staggering KO mountain in a style that overturns the common sense of boxing until then. Professional achievements, bouts 37 wins 36 KOs 31, lost only 1. WBC, WBO, IBF world featherweight champion with over 80% KO rate. His weapons are soft step work and weight shift (dive), accurate sense of distance, exceptional body sensation, and rhythm that make use of overwhelming momentary power. By observing the process to his KO with images, it shows a very interesting point. When standing and moving to the back side (in the case of the orthodox which is the left foot is at front, it is the left), he uses a fluffy step work. The opponent follows to that direction, trying to keep putting Hamed in his sight. Normally, except when consciously doing it, when a human follows the object to see, the eyes moves first then the body.

When Hamed is performing light steps to the left, the opponent's side moves his eyes→ then the body moves to the right.

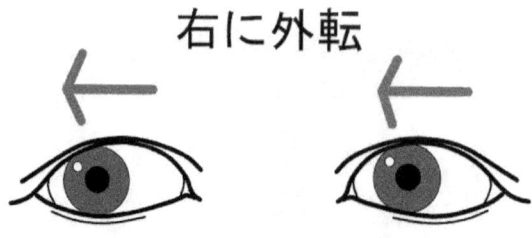

Hamed produces this flow with a step work to the side ... suddenly jumping forward and jumping like throwing his body weight and plunging, then slamming his punch on the opposite side. It seems that rather than a human being punching out, a feline animal like a leopard or a jaguar instantly kills his prey. The opponent's eyes have no time to be surprised because his eyes are forced to turn left and right, then receives his attack.

Humans try to secure safety by fixing the movement of the body while linking vision, equilibrium sense, and muscle output. For example, when an external force is applied, even if the Reflective function (vestibular ocular reflex) which tries to maintain the Visual information (visible landscape), or an external force applied to the brain disrupts the balance, the reflective function (vestibular neck reflex) which tries to restore to its original stable position, works as the system. When receive a strike while seeing it, these defensive reactions are easily come to work, and on the other hand, if you receive a strike while not seeing it, you gain difficulties for the defensive reactions. The fighters who was KOed by that, say "I didn't know what skill knocked me down" "I couldn't see the opponent's strike at all". On the other hand, even with a certain level of powerful attack, you will experience being able to bear without being overthrown if you get it in the state of seeing it and knowing it coming. The fighters whom were defeated, appeared they didn't know what happened right after they were knocked down. Like they "didn't see it coming". In addition, Hamed's punch uses a whole body like a soft spring, hits tackles by making full use of the jumping power, so "basic skill is body tackle" just like there is a glove on a part of it. So he can knockout either hand on the front or back, and even left and right he could do it. For those fighters who punches with the feet stopped, when seen from the opponent, only his gloves are being thrown, so it's easier to respond because the amount of the information from the eye sight is little. Since Hamed punches out with weight movement, so from the opponent's side, since multiple parts such as head, torso, pelvis, shoulder, and lower limbs come close simultaneously, the input amount of visual information on the retina becomes overwhelmingly more than the situation where only the glove blowing.

He is also a genius of controlling the rhythm. While he steps fluffily, comparatively slow rhythm. The opponent matches his rhythm subconsciously, like being forced to move by Hamed. The gentle comfortable rhythm comes without any precaution, suddenly modulates, cuts into you. It's like the elegant classical music suddenly turns into up-tempo hip-hop. He is an extraordinary fighter whom had produced surprises and defeated his opponents with such dramatic rhythmical change.

"Footwork tactics to control movement of the opponent's eyeball",
"KO punch delivered from all sides in front and back, left and right based on tackle",
"Control of the amount of information input to the opponent's vision",
"Radical rhythm change"

It is one of the role models beyond the era in which we can learn regardless.

1-6 【KO Training Method for Kicking】

Practicing using goods such as sandbags and mitts are very effective if you have a clear purpose, but if not, there are unexpected pitfalls. Because human beings are by no means conscious of being pulled our attention on the object or the environment in front of the eyes, so subconsciously the techniques become to be for sand bags and mitt.

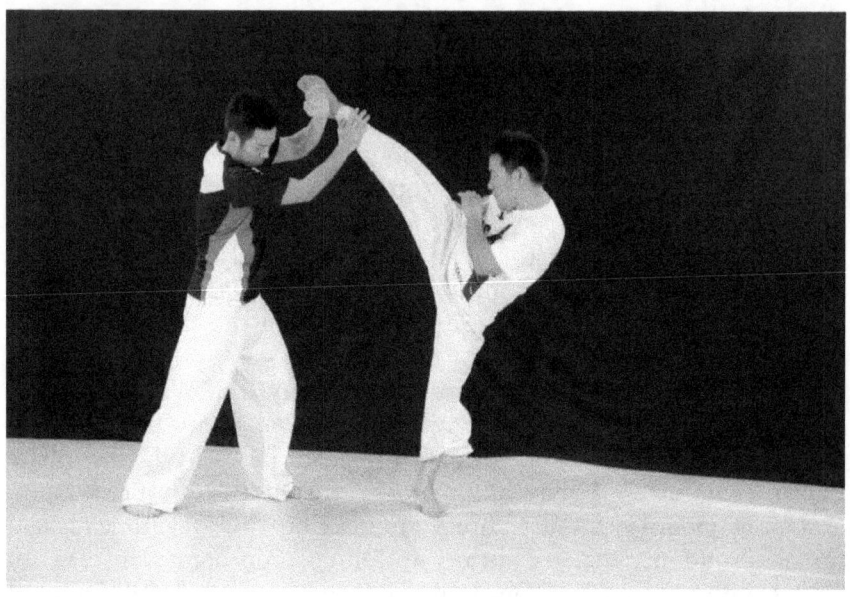

A world champion of strikes, was talking that the most important practice is "kicking the air" which you do not kick objects. "Before actually kicking, be sure to create the image in your head, as cutting the opponent sharply with your kick. Not just kicking without thinking, but go through the process of, Image→actual movement→fix the error, to do the "kicking the air" Otherwise it doesn't mean anything. As he said. Furthermore, "Grasp the moment that kicking hits, imagine up to the stage you knocked out your opponent. Never think of you can't do it, and kick as you can KO the opponent with it". As he spoke. However, if kicking 100 times without fixing anything, "number of times to improve" is zero. It was the secret of modern expert who creates KO, kicking the air that continues to make his improvements by making full use of the body and image in his brain.

1-7 【Real Grappler Baki's words】

Naoyuki Taira. Shoot boxing, K1, Vale-tudo, Jiu-Jitsu, martial arts, and so on, all riding in and out of all genres, rare existence beyond the genre barriers. He is famous as a model of fighting manga, Grappler Baki that is being read worldwide, and has inspired a lot of people. Mr.Taira and I got acquainted at the Maeda Hiroaki's professional fighting sports box office called "Rings", since then, has received tremendous cooperation in Fightology research activities and has advised as an advisor to the Society of Fighting Medicine At one point in the conversation with Mr. Taira, he told me

"It does not mean that the opponent gets knocked down with a strong blow, and if the opponent is knocked down with a weak blow, people will call it a strong blow"

I was shocked like getting a blow onto my brain. "If I don't Increase my body weight, and increase my body mass, to increase my power, I can't KO the opponent. The reason why I can't KO, is I don't give enough effort" Since I truly believed it at that time, I took the event called KO wrongly. Based on the words of Mr. Taira, I studied "What is KO?" from the medical aspect, and I examine it with practice and sparring. And I realized there is a very important thing. It turned out that the fighting sports and martial arts competition was a relationship between two people. Know yourself, know your opponent. And as the relationship goes on at the moment to moment between you and your opponent, you control yourself and lead the relationship. "Knocks down if a strong blow hits" is merely a belief of us, and is only expectation. Strong, weak, is only an evaluation of the surroundings. Mr. Taira made me realize that It is important to make a breakthrough "What is the strike which can KO".

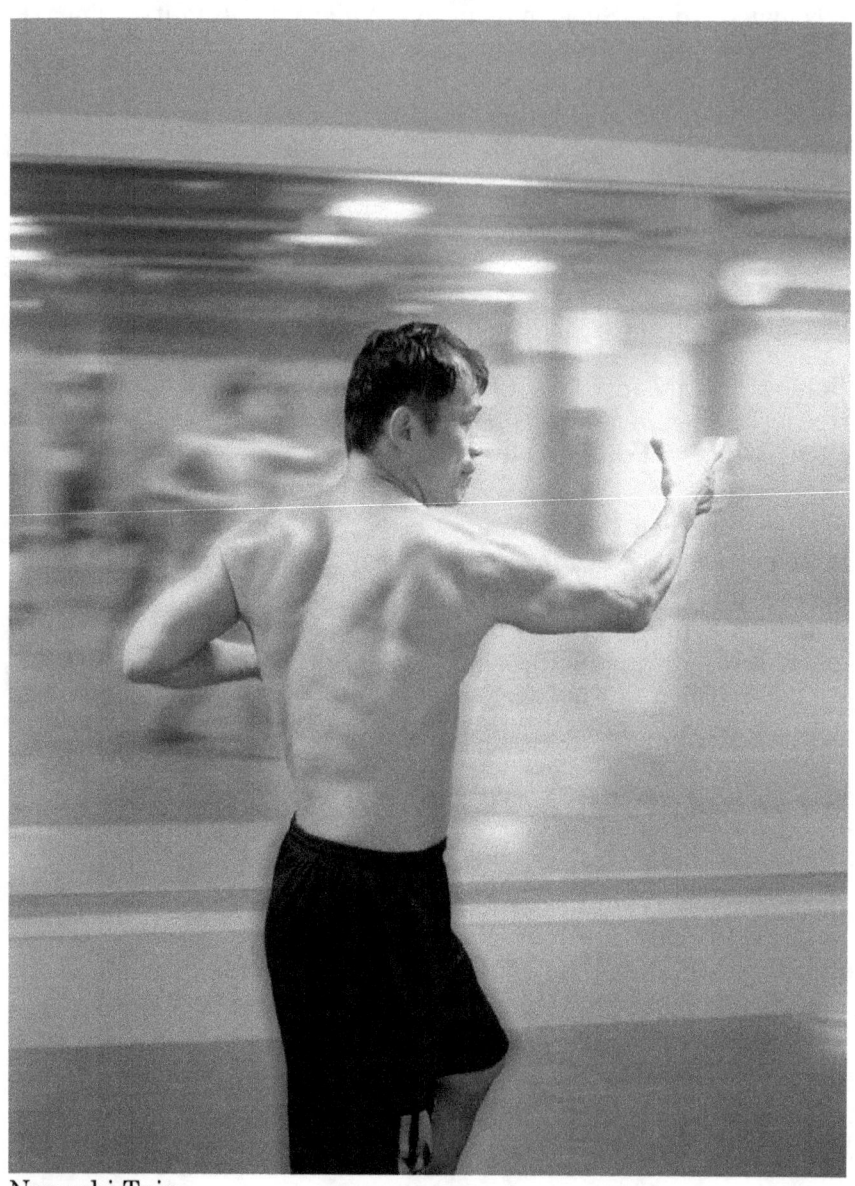

Naoyuki Taira

1-8 【Pinch turn over KO】

Excitement and pleasure when I KOed. It's not a lot of times, but I also experienced KO victory during the time of me as a fighter. It is an overwhelming feeling that you can not taste in other things. The stronger your opponent, the harder it is during the match and the more likely the heart breaks, the more KO will settle as an unforgettable memory. That's the condition that the endorphin is produced in the brain. I tell the story to the fighters that KO is "Do you know what is the abbreviation for KO? It's K (Kamisamano = the god's, in Japanese) O (Okurimono = gift, in Japanese)[which comes "A gift from a god]". KO is a result at last, there seems to be a gift for a person who carefully accumulated the process of trial and error leading to it. Rather than just asking for KO, "reproducibility" may be established on the precision and persistence like craftsmen who carefully create the situation where KO comes down from above. KO, especially reversal KO, is nothing other than turning the pinch over. The confidence you can get there can be enormous and permanent. Even when there are unreasonable things in real life, even when if you encounter a wall and you are about to give up, if you imagine "linking to the situation of yourself "How to reverse KO from this situation?" from the experience of your match, somehow you may see the light. Is not such experience a wonderful benefit of fighting sports and martial arts?

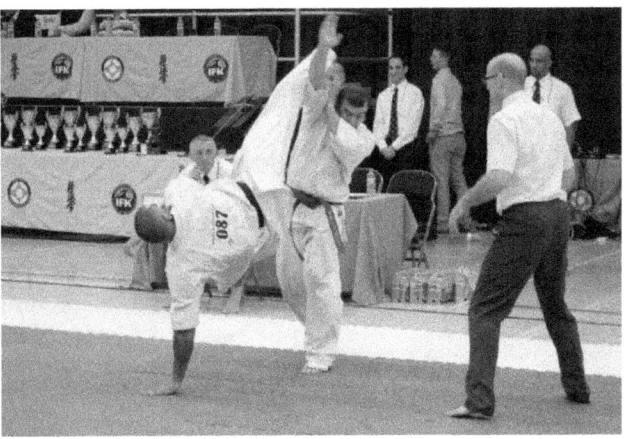

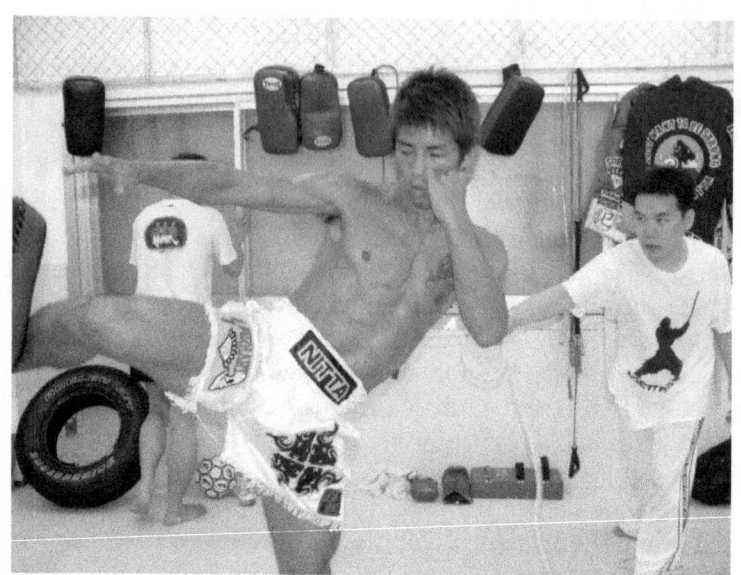

Training with Kickboxing world champ, Nitta Akeomi

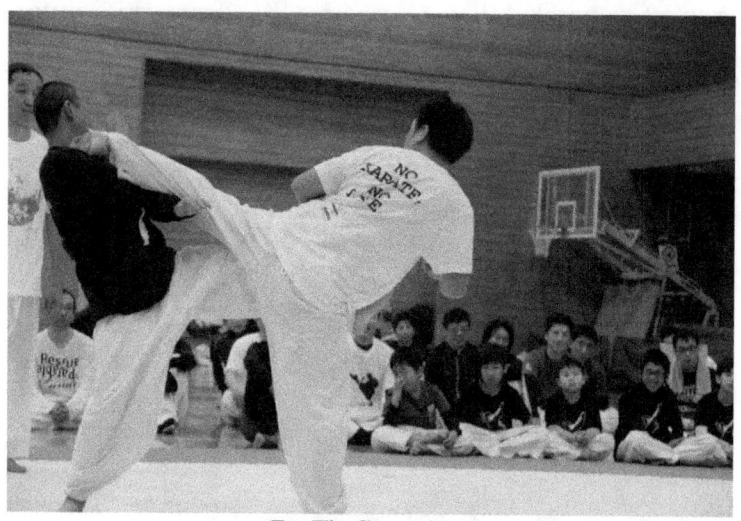

Dr.F's Sparring

2:WHAT IS KO?
-BODY-

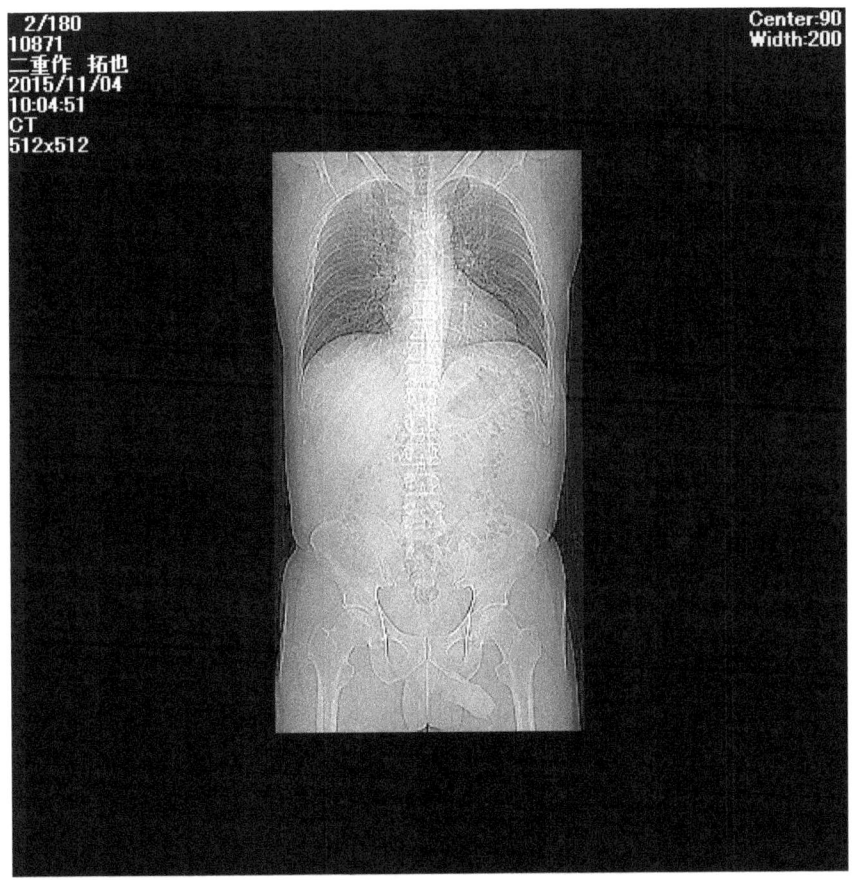

2-1 【KO with body blow】

Speaking of the KO scenes in fighting sports, I think that many people on the watching side think of players falling down due to punching and kicking techniques to the face. KO in the attack on the face is also aware of the consciousness, and it is "flashy" so there is some sort of "easy to know what happened". However, if you step forward from the "viewer side" to the "doing side" to repeatedly practice and fighting the matches, you could actually feel how high level technic it is, about the meaning of body attacks, and how to make the body blows effective with a single punch or kick.

When being knocked down by attack on the face, since the consciousness disappears transiently, it is in a state of "fallen down when I noticed", and the memory of being knocked down does not remain. On the other hand, the KO with the body blows, as compared with that on the face, the process remained in memory, the one who loses will win "complete defeat", and the winner will taste" complete victory ". KO with body blows which is "being not able to move with consciousness remained clear". Let's explore the mechanism.

完全決着

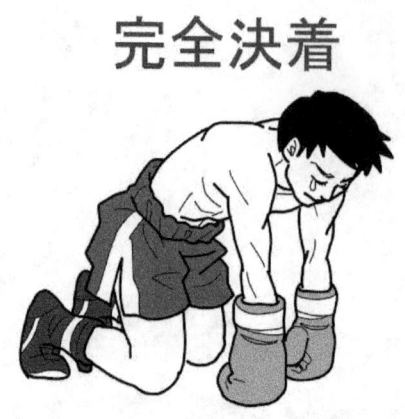

42

2-2 【We don't feel pain on the liver or the stomach itself】

In fighting sports and martial arts, attacks on internal organs such as liver, epigastrium (stomach) and spleen are effective, and even in boxing they call it liver blow, and in Karate they call it liver uchi(hit). In fact, if you get to that part properly, you may "Ugh" then it will make you almost stop breathing, and you will feel a heavy and dull pain over the abdomen. This is a distinctive sensation of pain that is totally different from pain when you get hit on muscles and joints. I myself have experienced a lot of times, the effectiveness of the body loses willingness to fight, and I do not want to move any further. When damage is great, we strike along with sweat. If a "slap" that puts you in the fighting spirit was a "body blow", the fighting spirit will surely disappear.

When the time I was a medical intern, I had a very interesting incident when I was training in the anesthesiology department. The anesthesiologist is mainly responsible for monitoring the heart rate, respiration rate, blood pressure and so on while managing the whole body of the patient, while creating a condition to for surgeons to perform surgery with concentration. Since the surgery cuts the tissue with a scalpel, if the general anesthesia is ineffective, the heart rate jumps up, and in some cases the patient moves and that is a danger, so the anesthesiologist controls the situation when the heart rate is likely rising by increasing the concentration of aesthetic gas and giving injections. At the removal of liver cancer, the surgeon cuts out the parenchyma of the liver containing cancer cells and removes it. I had a real experience (was it a prejudice?) that "That's an efficient pain when I hit a liver or an internal organs!" I was preparing by anticipating that the heart rate would rise when the scalpel cut the parenchyma of the liver. However, this did not rise more than my expectation. I felt somewhat I was fooled, but at that time I remembered with "Argh" it was a medical knowledge that "the internal organs themselves are not easy to feel pain." The liver cells constituting the liver has high regenerative ability and is not easy to feel pain, so the liver is called "mute organ" or "silent organ". Even if the parenchyma of the liver is actually cut with a scalpel during surgery such as liver tumor, the patient does not feel pain much. Also, there is no sensory receptor for pain in the stomach and intestine itself. Therefore, even if you cut or hurt by surgery, it is less likely to feel pain. It is when "the function got worse" that the stomach and intestines hurt. When the stomach hurts due to the nervousness before the match, the muscles around the stomach will shrink and the pain will be transmitted to the brain. Moreover, when you feel your stomach hurts because after eating too much, you will feel pain due to your stomach expanding. Mm? It is strange. Even though there is no sense of pain in the liver, in the stomach nor in the intestine, why is it so painful when you get a strike on the abdomen? One that holds the key is the tissue called "peritoneum".

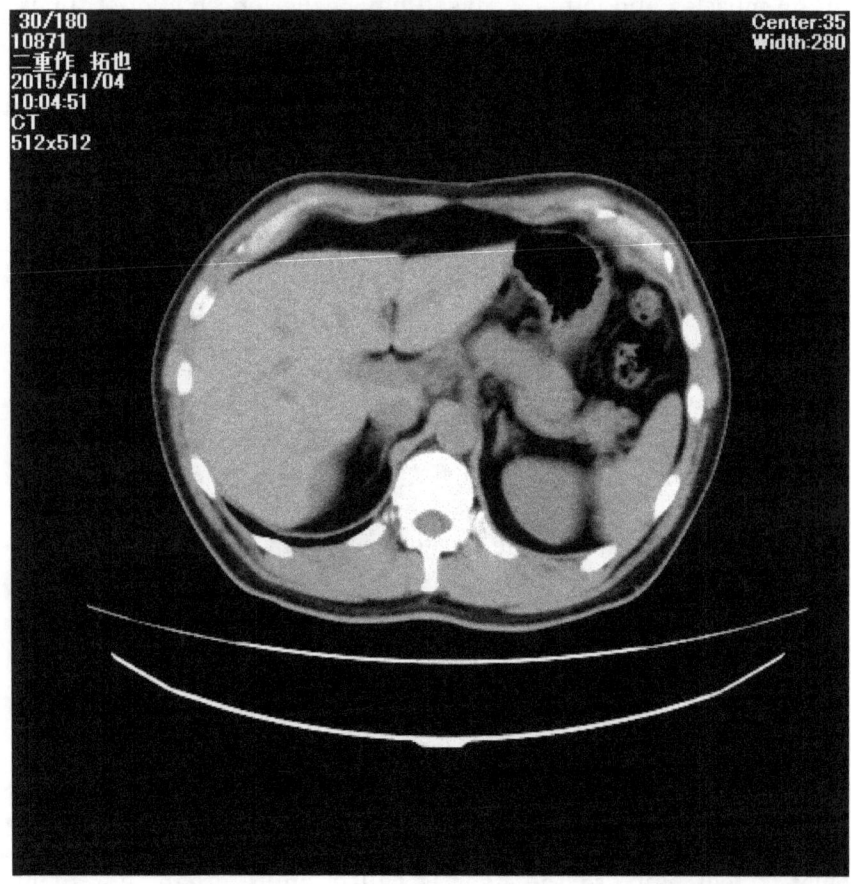

2-3 【KO and peritoneum】

Peritoneum is a thin semitransparent membrane that covers the abdominal organs such as stomach, intestines, liver and so on. There is a lot of pain sense on this peritoneum, we feel strong pain when stimulated. It is thought that the reason why being hit on epigastrium is that effective, is organ covering "peritoneum" gets pain stimulation. The pain experienced with liver strike is not the pain of the liver itself but is the pain that the peritoneum which covers the liver felt. For men folks, hasn't anyone had once or twice the experience of hitting hard vulnerable part(testicles) and writhed in pain? After a little moment you get hit, your lower abdomen becomes strikingly heavy, sigh like "Ugh" which isn't really a voice comes out, then cold sweat drips... It is not easy for women to sympathize with this pain, but being honest, I feel sick just by writing it (sweat). The pain of being hit on testicle and the pain when you get a body blow are similar in kind. The testicles are originally the ovaries of women. In the early days of the fetus, it is in the abdominal cavity, but it steadily gets down and fills in the bag. Since the testicles are also one of internal organs, they are covered with the peritoneum. Furthermore, it is more sensitive to pain than the internal organs because it is densely covered with a tissue called tunica albuginea testis which is also a pain sensory receptor. Oops, every woman who is reading this, you should not try your "groin kick" to your husband or boyfriend! The pain you feel in skin and muscle is called "somatic pain", the pain you feel by being stimulated to the internal organs and its surroundings called "visceral pain", but comparing with somatic pain is clear in the area of pain, the scope is also limited, the visceral pain, whereas the part of pain is unclear, while the range is also unclear. Because somatic pain and visceral pain differ in the route that the pain stimulus reaches the brain, even the same pain causes such a difference. Even in fighting sports and martial arts, when the low kick is kicked out and it is effective, the part kicked is painful, but when the body blow is made effective, wider than the part being hit, whole abdomen gets the pain spread "whump!" with discomfort after a little while.

2-4 【Body structure and protection】

Next, let's think about how to make the strikes reach the peritoneum easier, from the aspect of the abdominal structure. If we talk about the structure of the body (abdomen), the most outside surface is the skin, then the subcutaneous tissue, and there are abdominal muscles in the end. The group of abdominal muscles consists of rectus abdominis muscle, outer oblique muscle, inner oblique muscle and transverse abdominal muscles, and the peritoneum is even deeper than these abdominal muscles. Since the internal organs are important tissues / organs for human to live, if they are injured by external injuries, that risks our lives! So that's why it's naturally "protected" by a tough group of abdominal muscles. Even you attack the body, at that moment, if your opponent's muscles contract strongly, you will not be able to stimulate his/her peritoneum adequately as it is being blocked by muscle walls.

Even ordinary people are made to contract against pain stimulations, so it is not easy to make the body of fighting sport fighters and martial artists with well trained thick abdominal muscles groups. However, top fighters have their respective expertise to make the body blows work. Whether consciously or unconsciously, "a state where abdominal muscle group is difficult to contract," or strategically create "a situation where abdominal muscle group is difficult to contract" to establish a path to KO.

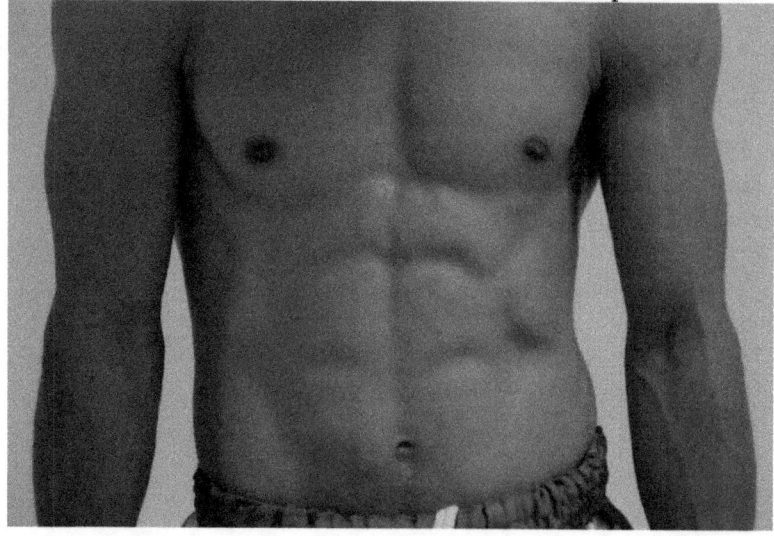

2-5 【KO strategy ~double strike, triple strike~】

There is a nature that muscles can not sustain the maximum shrinkage for a long time. Think of the hanging from the steel bar and raising yourself to the top with suspension. No matter how powerful you are, you will lose by the gravity sometime as time goes on. This is because the muscles that contract when raised up can not sustain the contraction for a single impulse. It's the same case for abdominal muscle group.

Even if it can be strongly contracted for a moment, it is impossible to maintain the maximum contraction state for a long time. In the fighting sports, when you receive the first blow, even if you strongly contract the group of abdominal muscles to maximum and endure the attack on the body, if you get the second hit soon afterwards, the muscle contraction drops down seamlessly. Therefore, even if you hit the second and subsequent blows with the same strength as the first one, the stimulation to the peritoneum will increase. Fighter who is good at body attacks is skillfully using this property and makes the opponent to shrink the abdominal muscle group on purpose on the first hit, then with the timing when it start being loose, then gives second and third hit, to let the stimulation reaches to the peritoneum. If the interval between the first and second is too large, the contraction of the maximum tension occurs more easily, so we will aim the timing of the muscle contraction ratio drops. In the full contact Karate system where punching to the face is prohibited, the technology of KO with the body blow is well developed.

Some fighter is good at a tactic that to keep punching the opponent's body constantly to make the body blows work. That fighter told me the secret that the tip is as light attack as letting the opponent thinks "It doesn't work". The strategy of how to lower the protection effect of the abdominal muscles, is the tactic of double strike, triple strike.

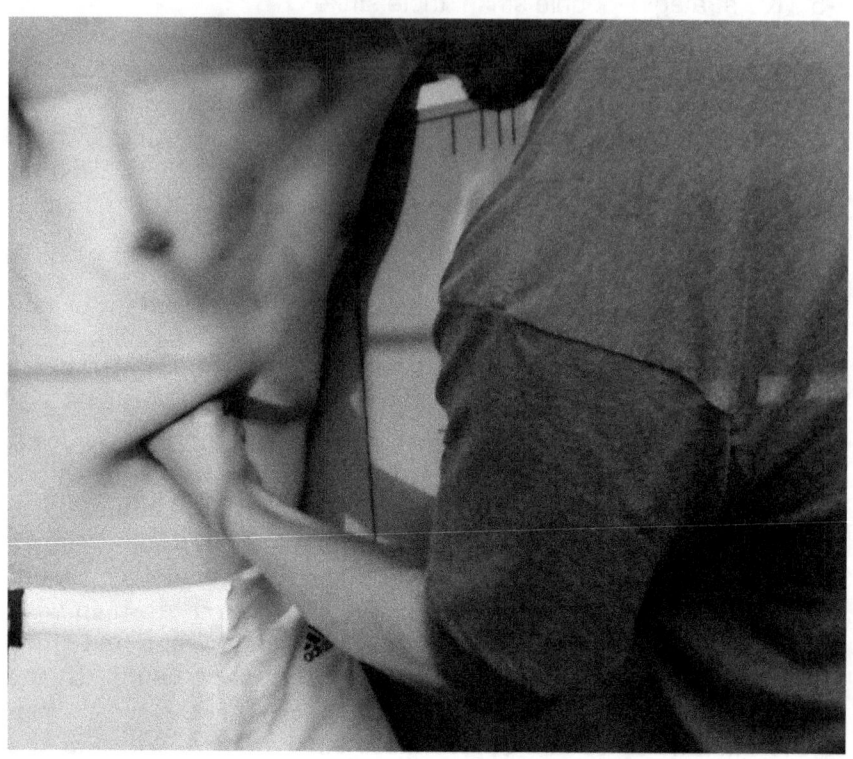

2-6 【Attack of a pain on surface, attack reaching deep place】

Have you ever seen a performance demonstration such as "beating with a bat or a square lumber on the stomach" of Karate or martial arts? Outside the worry of the audience that "Are the internal organs okay with being struck with such a hard thing?", the performers keep their countenance.

When the human's abdomen is damaged and stimulated on the body surface, at the instance the muscle is connected with it so as to shrink strongly. At this moment, the muscles become walls of the peritoneum and internal organs and protected, so the stimulation to the internal organs and their surroundings is smaller than the size of the sound and the gaudy appearance. Of course, the reason why the Karatekas and martial artists can do such a performance is because the abdominal muscles are thick, be able to reduce the damage, and they can consciously use the abdominal muscles intentionally as a protector. It is a gift from the accumulation of consistent trainings, and if a person who does not train tries to do it, it will be a big mess.

By the way, when you were a child, was there any experience of getting groaned when relatively soft objects such as soccer balls and volleyball hit your stomach? When a thing that is soft or a thing which doesn't hurt even if it hits, hits the abdomen, the pain stimulation to the body surface is little, so the muscles tend to be strongly resistant to shrinkage. As a result, if it is a soft object, on the contrary it is difficult to protect the internal organs and the peritoneum. When you get a massage, when a skilled massager touches softly, the muscle remains relaxed, so stimulation is pleasant and there is a feeling that the stimulation reaches deep inside, but when a unskilled massager pushes hard strongly, muscles become rigid and be caught in pain and only discomfort increases and the body may not accept it anymore of it. Like this case, the pain stimulus and the muscle tension are closely related. When attacking the body with a punch, when you strike hard with a hard fist from the beginning, it may encourage contraction of the muscles of the abdomen, and stimulation may be difficult to reach the peritoneum.

A fighter who thinks "I should hit hard with a strong stuff" is said to be "it is not effective even I hit this much" → "I have to put more power" → "I am hitting with strong power so it consumes stamina" tends to fall into such a loop.As a prescription to such fighters, at the moment of hitting the surface, keep the fist soft without grasping the fist tightly yet, and correct the timing to grasp where the fist went in deeply. Doing so makes the peritoneum more susceptible to stimulate and makes it easier to damage with body attacks.

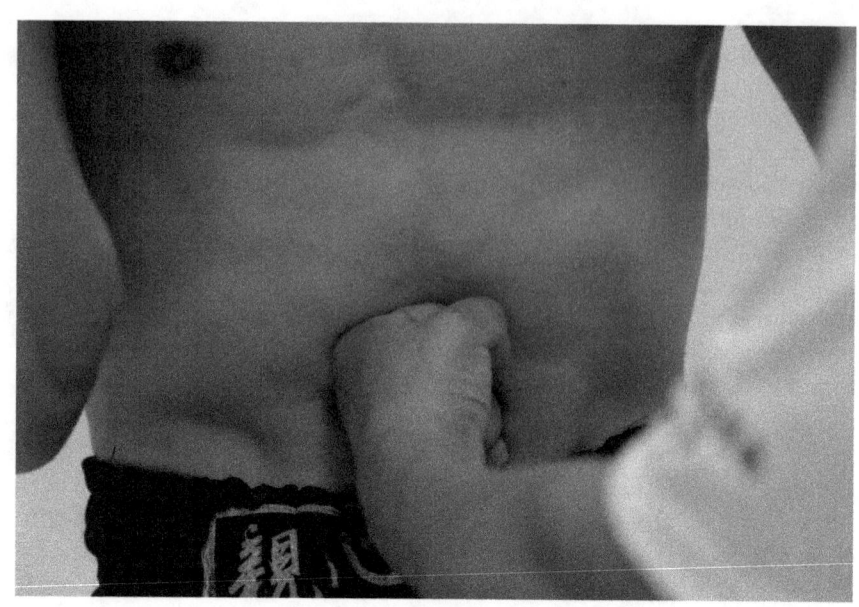

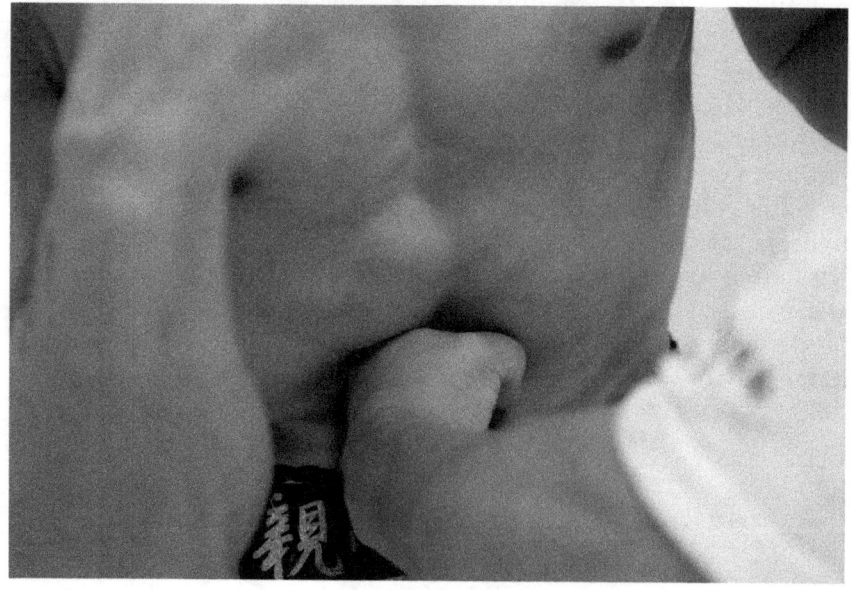

2-7 【A strike of shifting the part to hit】

A strike of shifting the place to hit is also effective for body blow KO. At the very first moment, the muscle group of the hit part contracts strongly, but there is also a technique to devise a strike so that power is applied to the part far from there at the next moment. In the case of a punch with bare hands, instead of hitting a knuckle part (MP joint) right away, one method is to put the joint on the distal part (fingertip part) first on the abdomen and subsequently apply the MP joint is an effective method as well. That is, although it is one punch, but there are two strikes to two parts. By shifting the place to hit, stimulation can be applied to the part where the contractile force has decreased.

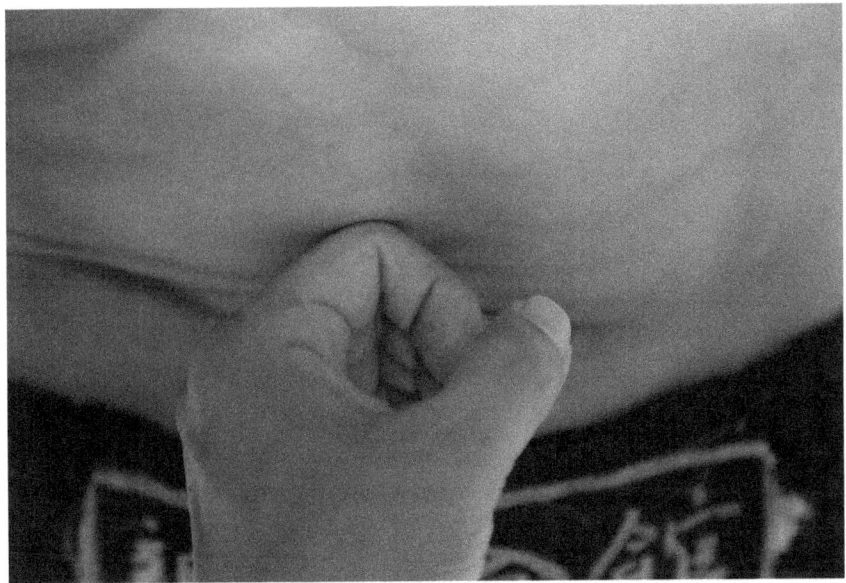

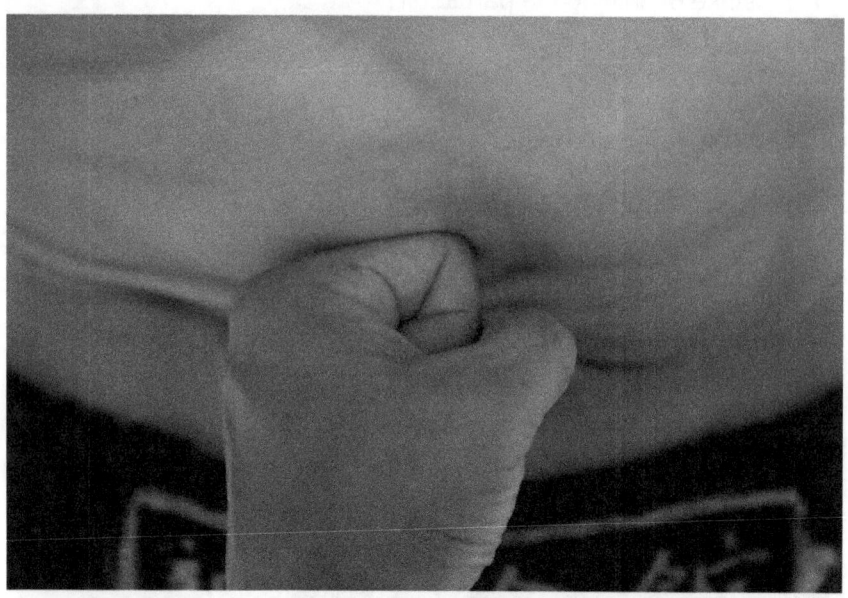

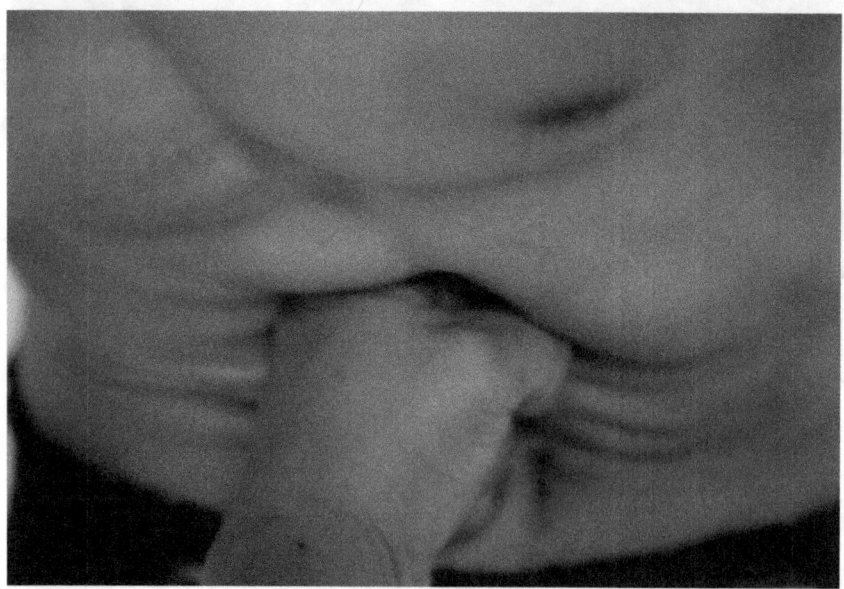

The strike of shifting part to is effective even for hitting gloves and open finger gloves used in mixed martial arts as well. The moment the glove hits the abdomen of the opponent, do not press on with the same surface, but change the hitting part slightly to hit, the one whom took it in might get a bigger damage. Also, with a body punch at a mount position of mix martial arts, it is effective to use different points of hitting without striking at the surface as well. The viewpoint of how to use gloves and open finger gloves in competition, is the area where it is worth to research, as there are a lot of fighters who are not conscious.

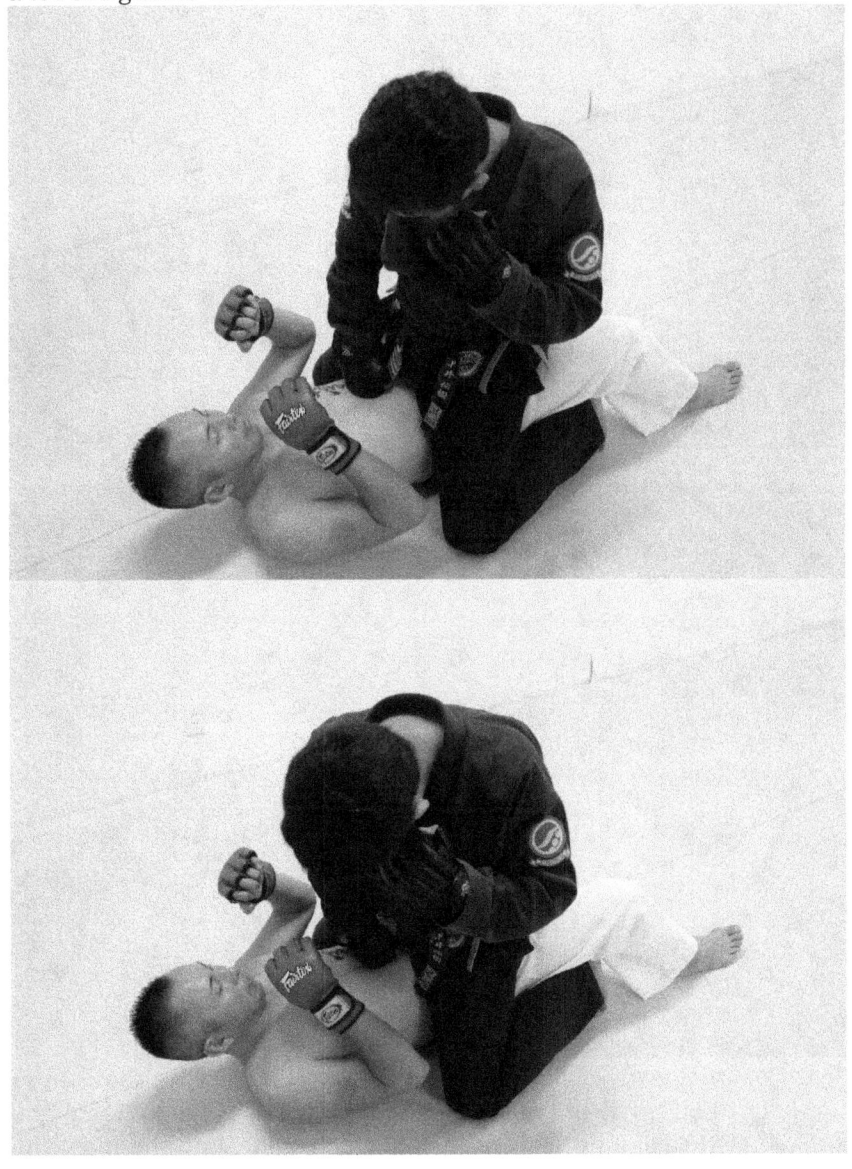

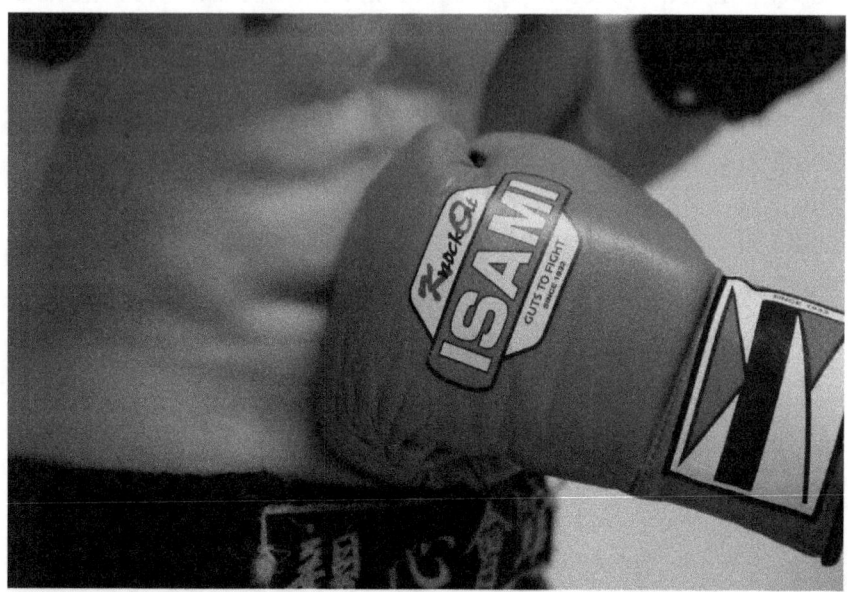

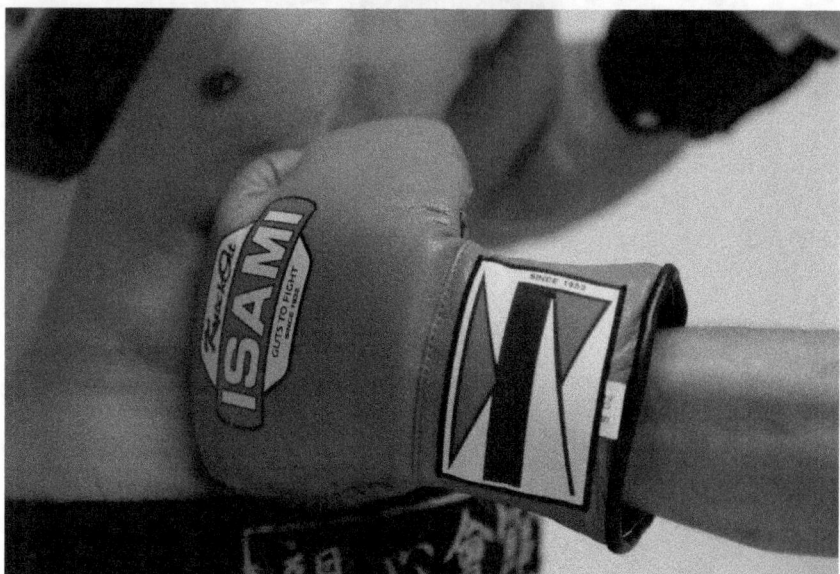

Even in the case of kicking into the body, a strike that shifts the part to be hit is effective. At the moment of knee kicking, the knee joint flexes, planter flexion of the foot joint, and the toes (the fingers of the feet) are bent, the patella (the bones of the knee plate) is displaced in the direction of the lower thigh. Even for front kicks and back kicks, there are methods that make it easier for damage to reach the deep part while using each joint well. Within the safe range where there are no injuries and damage remaining, the time to pursue a better way with a trustworthy practice fellow is "It's not that, it's not this" and the time to pursue a good method is a fun thing even you would forget the time runs even in practice.

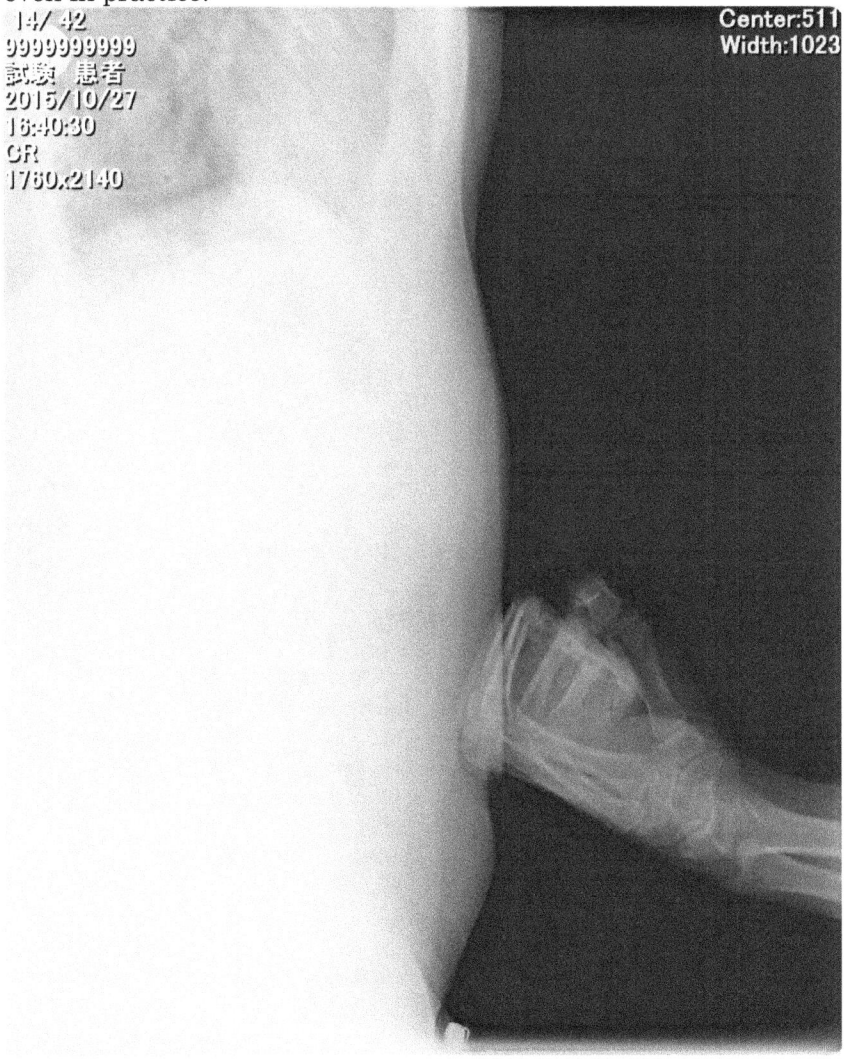

(Hard fist)

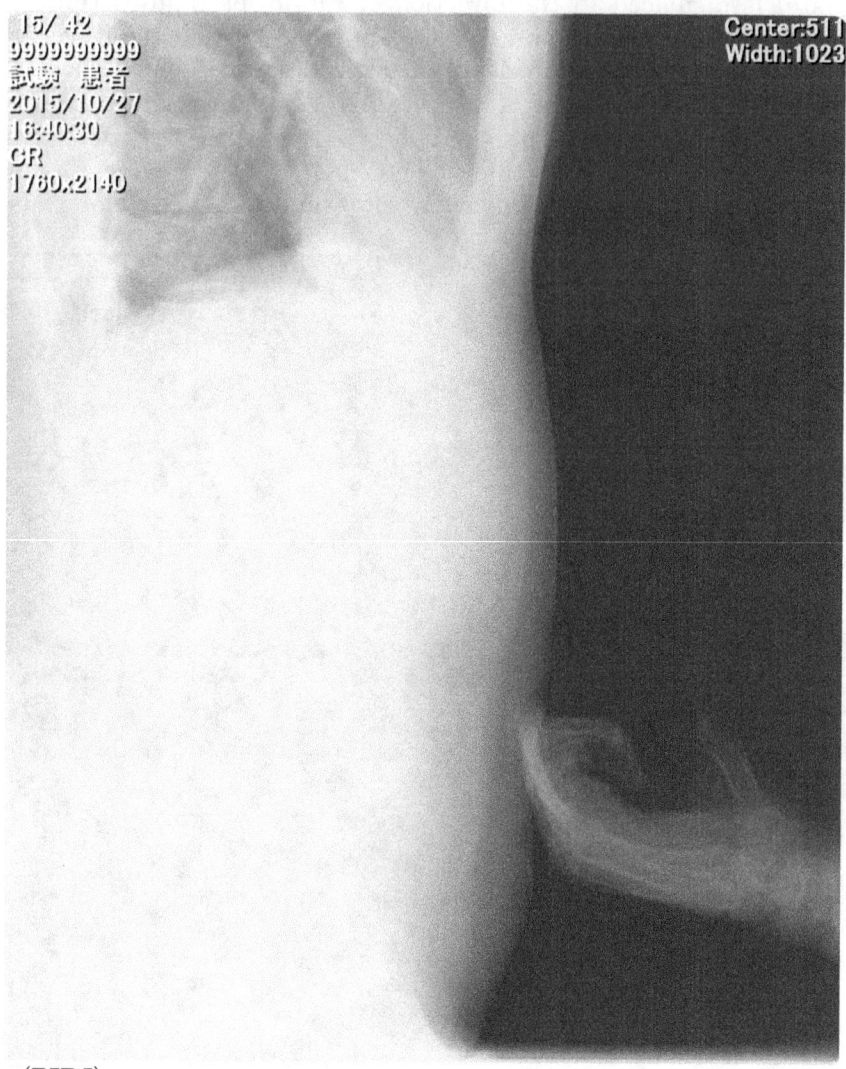

(PIPJ)

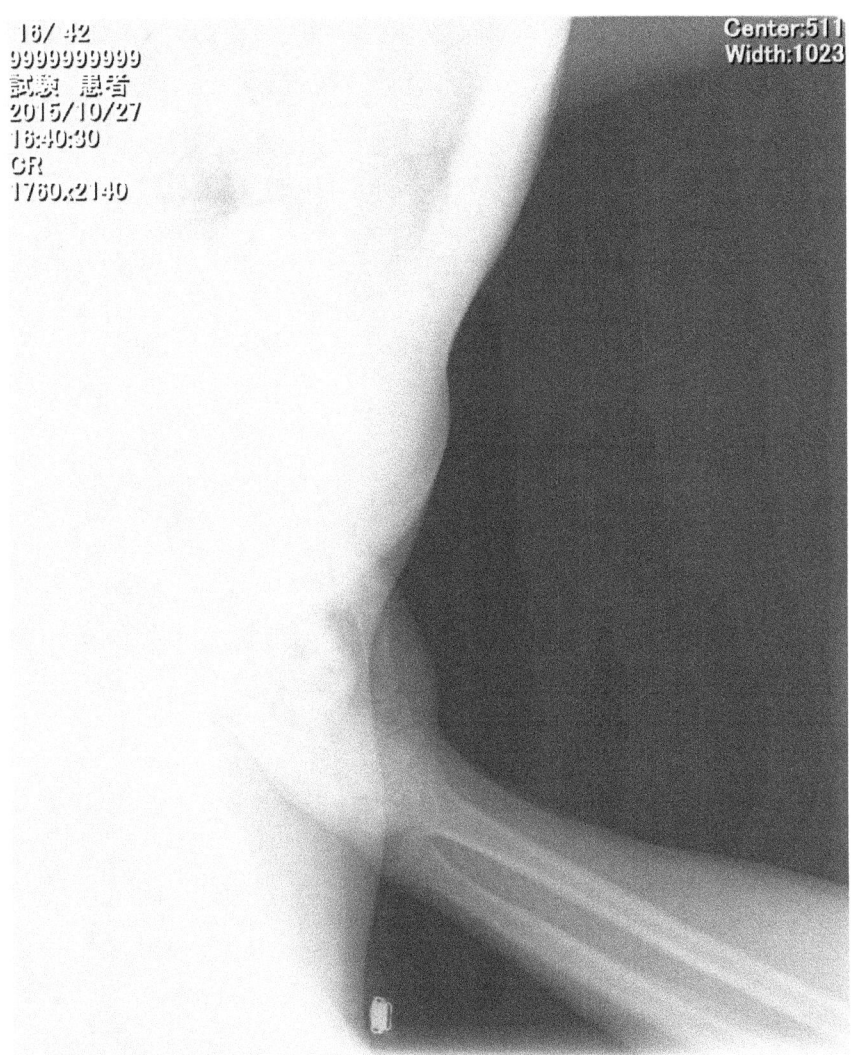

（MPJ go inside）

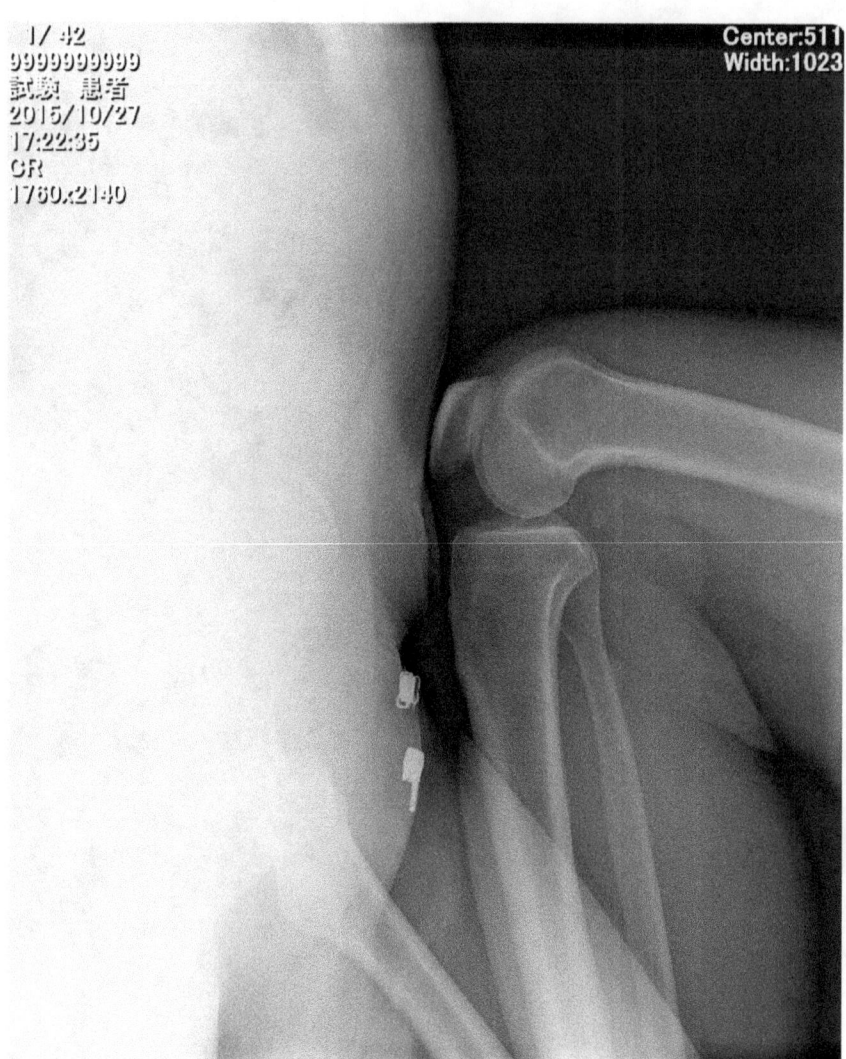

(Knee Kick 1)

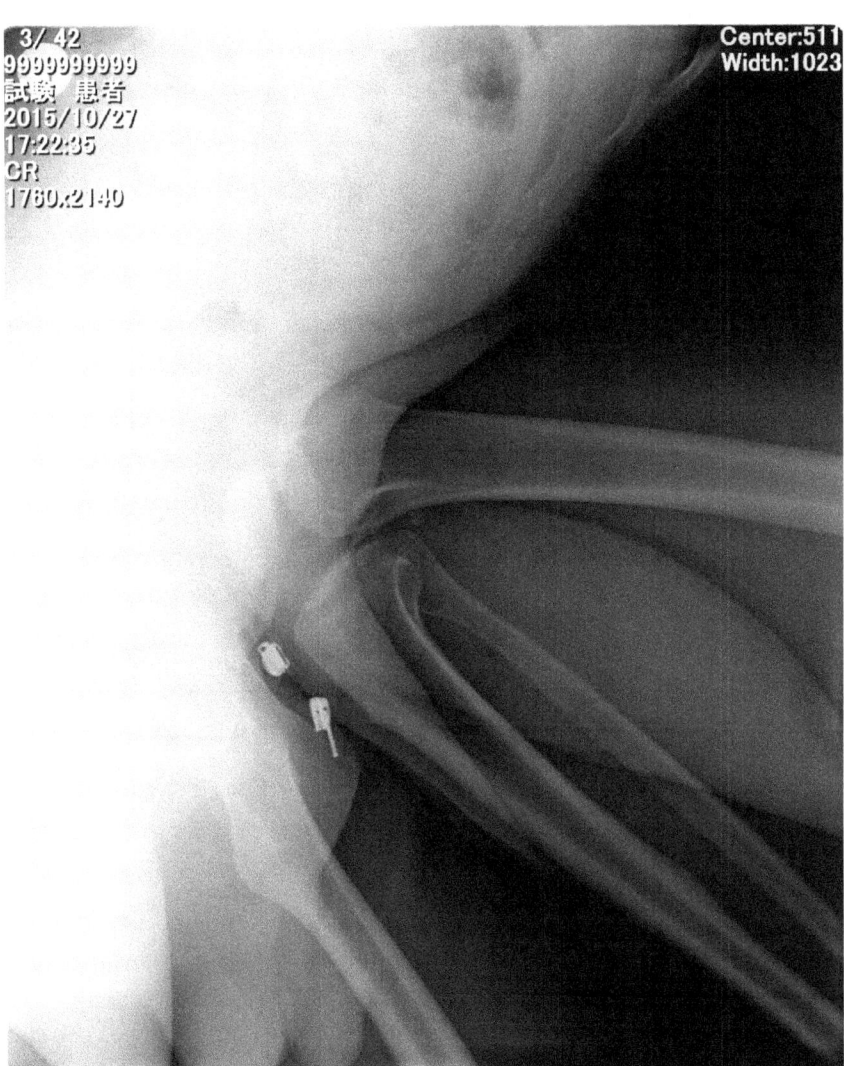

(Knee Kick 2)

2-8 【Breathing and body attack】

This time, let's do a simple experiment to know the relationship between breathing and the body blow. Make a partner, then

A: Get a punch on your body while inhaling.
B: Get a punch on your body while holding your breath
C: Get a punch on your body while exhaling.

What happens if you try these 3 patterns and arrange them in order of which is greater damage? (Please stay safe and without injury!) Even though the punch is the same strength, the damage of the receiver is totally different. The answer is A, B, C in order of ranking. Getting hit while breathing in is the biggest damage, if you get hit anyway, getting hit while breathing out, is the least damage. Let's think about this mechanism.

Below the lungs, there is a diaphragm that plays an important role in respiration. The diaphragm is mainly made of muscles and has a convex dome shape on the top. We often see "Harami" in Japanese yakiniku restaurant, Harami is a diaphragm of a beef cow. When the diaphragm contracts, the vertex of the diaphragm that was convex upwards comes down and the dome becomes low. With that, since the negative pressure is applied to the outside of the lung above the dome, the lungs can enlarge itself to breathe in. Below the diaphragm, there is an internal organ. As the diaphragm goes down, the space of the abdominal cavity containing the internal organs becomes smaller. So when you breathe in and get hit on your body, there is no escape place for abdominal organs. As a result, the body blow gets effective. Conversely, even if you get hit when you are breathing out like the case C, the diaphragm will relax and go up, so the internal escape space will be larger than the case A. Even if you get hit on your body at that time, it is hard to be effective.

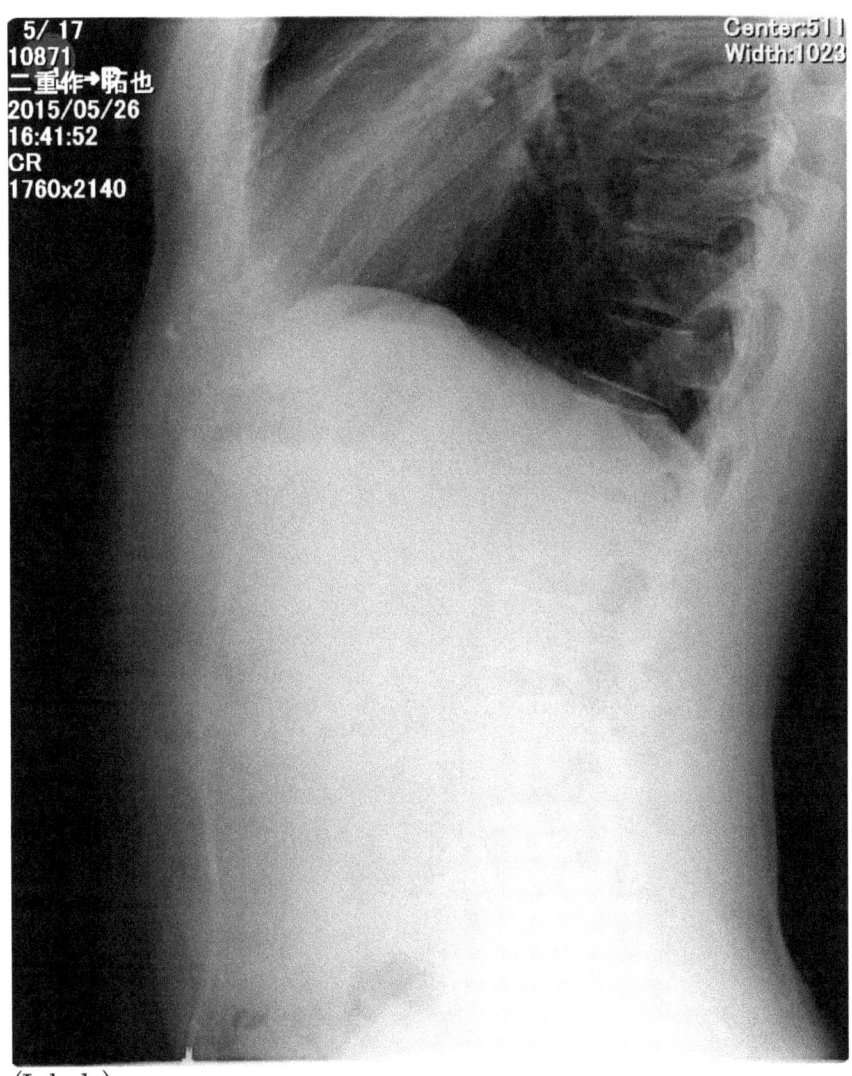

(Inhale)

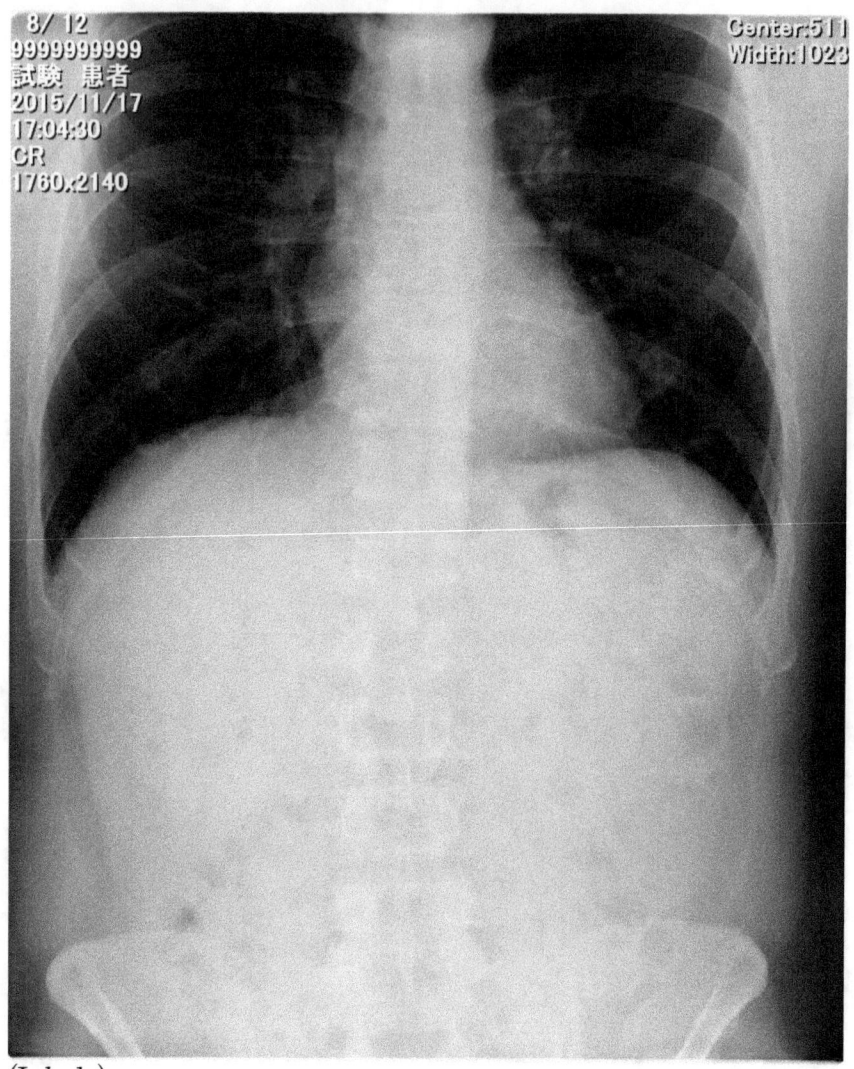

(Inhale)

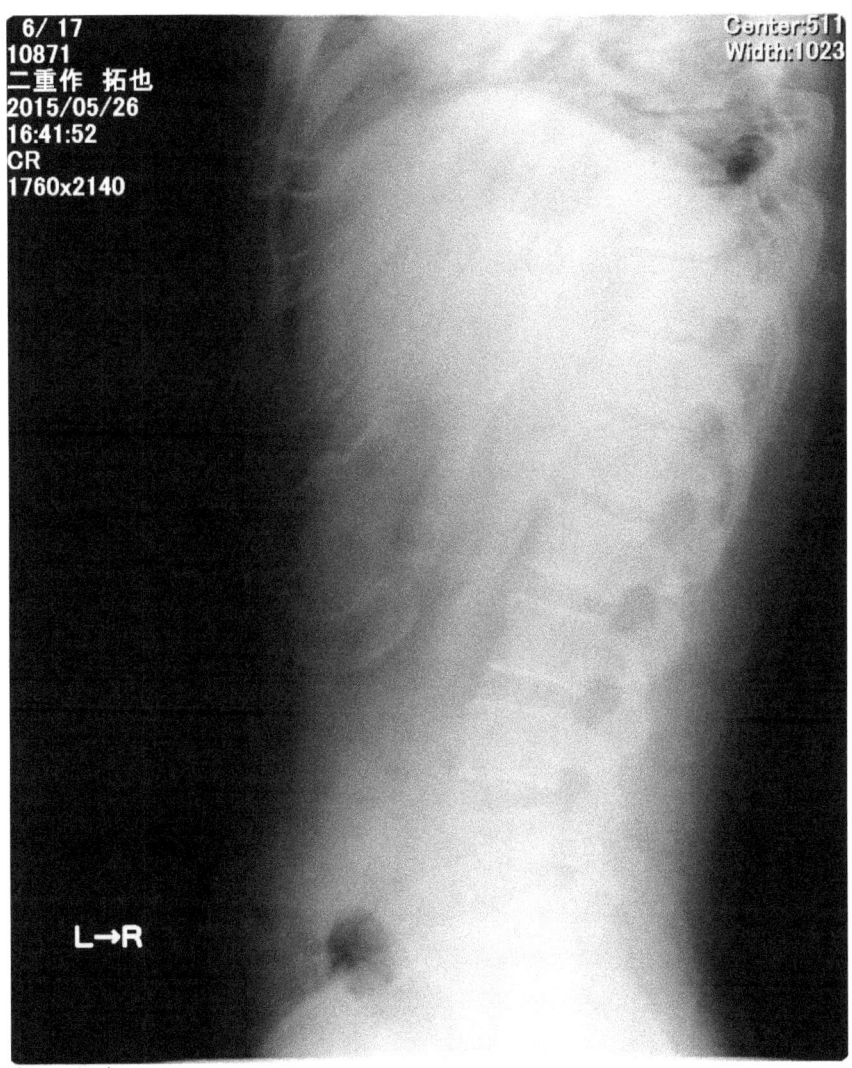

(Exhale)

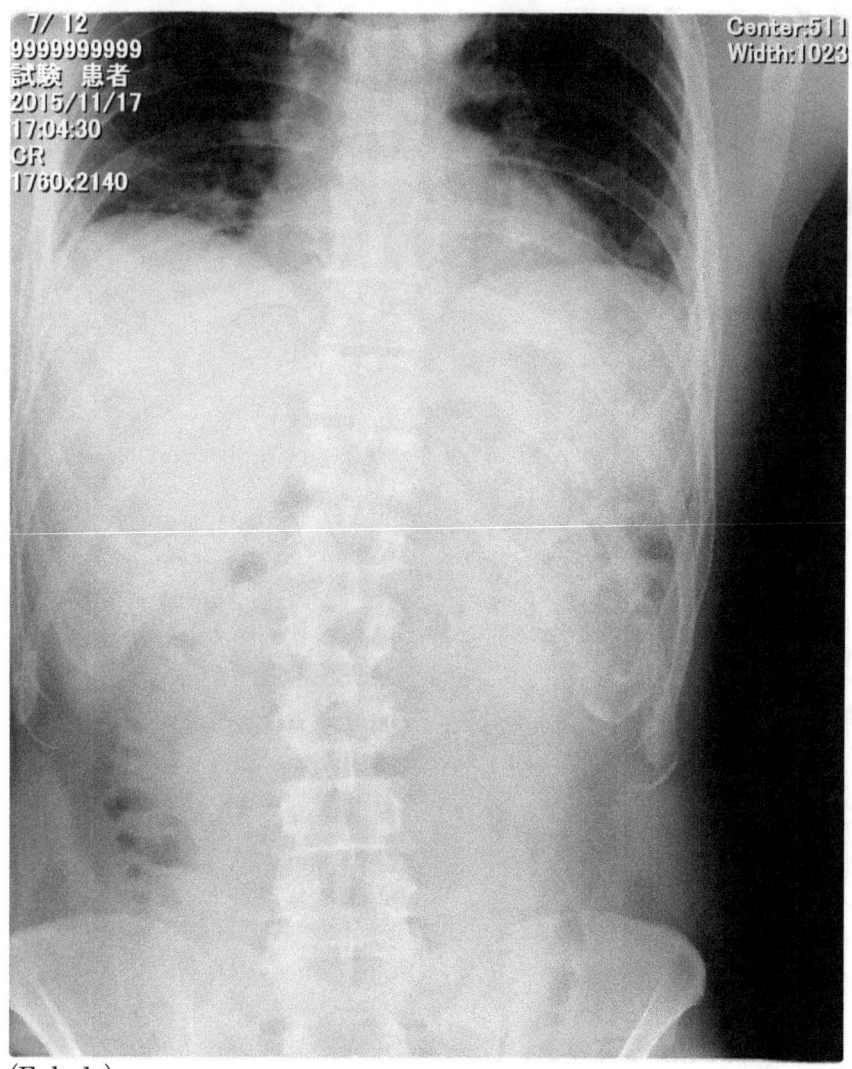

(Exhale)

Does a player who is weak of being hit on his/her body, stop breathing or take a long time to breathe in during the match? One of the breathing methods traditionally transmitted in Karate is "Ibuki". Inhale with a short moment, exhale slowly while fully moving the stomach and diaphragm, and finally breath out all the air. From a medical point of view, it seems like the message that the breath hurts "the breath-taking time should be made as short as possible and you should move while breathing" is hidden inside. The fighters whom are good at body strikes do not miss the timing when opponents breathe in. In the world of martial arts, it is sometimes referred to as "reading breath", but the ability to read breathing of the opponent appearing in motion is also a skill that will be useful in progressing body attacks.

2-9 【What moment is breathing in? 】

So what is the moment when you breathed in? Even if you were told "Hit at the moment when the opponent is breathing in!", Even if your opponent breathes "I breathed in now", "I breathed out now," and there is a lamp on the head and it lights up to tell so, it will be very helpful, but I can not hope for such a mechanism like a comedy show. We medical doctor, how we will look to check the patient's breathing during surgery, is to see if "the chest is moving or not". It is judged that there is breathing when the chest is moving, but since the partner is moving during the match and in the sparrings, you say "Please let me check breath for a moment" to ask to stop it for that purpose. If you say at every sparring "Excuse me, show me your chest a little while" to the female fighters, there will be a decision for you being a pervert champion in the dojo (cold sweat).

So how are top players reading the opponent's breaths? Also, how do you become able to read your opponent's breath? I myself had been concerned since when I was a fighter. Even if I was told "Read the breath", I could not understand what it means "reading breath" in the movements of the sparring. Although I learned the method to see it by looking at the shoulder, it is certain that the stamina is running out due to extension or re-extension, there are times when the state of breathing heavily on the shoulder appears, but when the stamina is still running well in the main battle, it is difficult for change to appear on the shoulder, and it is hard for a fighter with a career has the skill to trick your eyes, so I felt is is difficult to follow that method.

"How can I read breath?" I had been asking myself, and the hint was in a surprising place. It was music. There is a small V character on the score when singing a song. It is a sign called "Breath" which signifies "Please breathe in here." To sing a song is to exhaling while making a voice, so at the end of a phrase there is always a moment to breathe. When putting out a skill in a match, there are times when you set a combination, such as "one - two - right low" "left jab to right middle". These are the phrases in the song. At the final blow of the combination after invoking "Sh" "Heh" etc. there certainly is going to have "breath". If you strike the body securely at this moment, damage will be very large even if the punch is the same strength. A combination of "one - two, right - low" comes with a chance of body attack right after the right-low. To hit the body and make it effective, I think that if you put in a habit of catching the "break of movement" linked with "break of breath", that success rate surely increases.

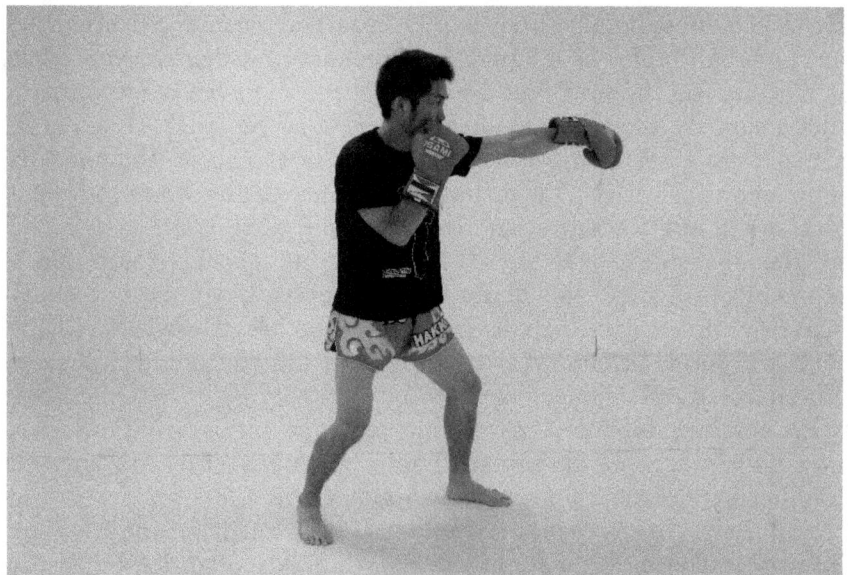

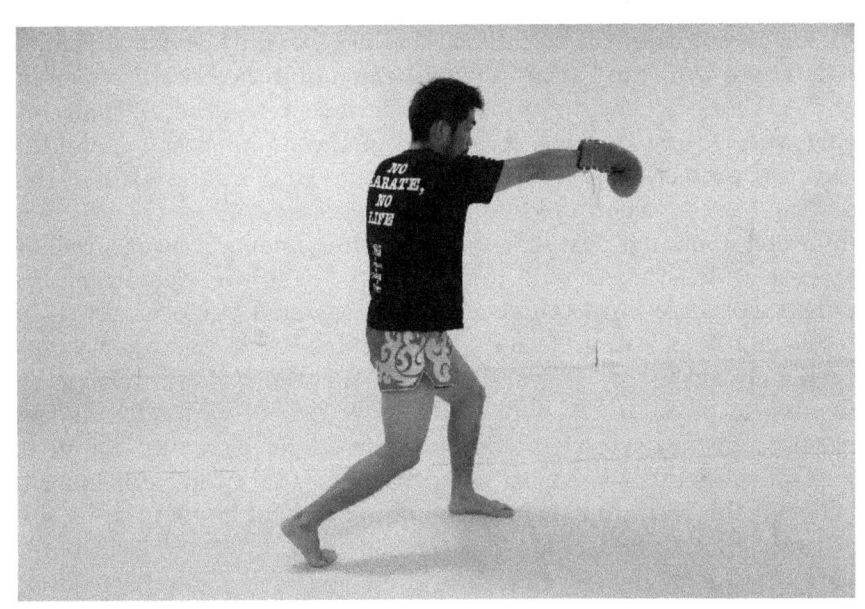

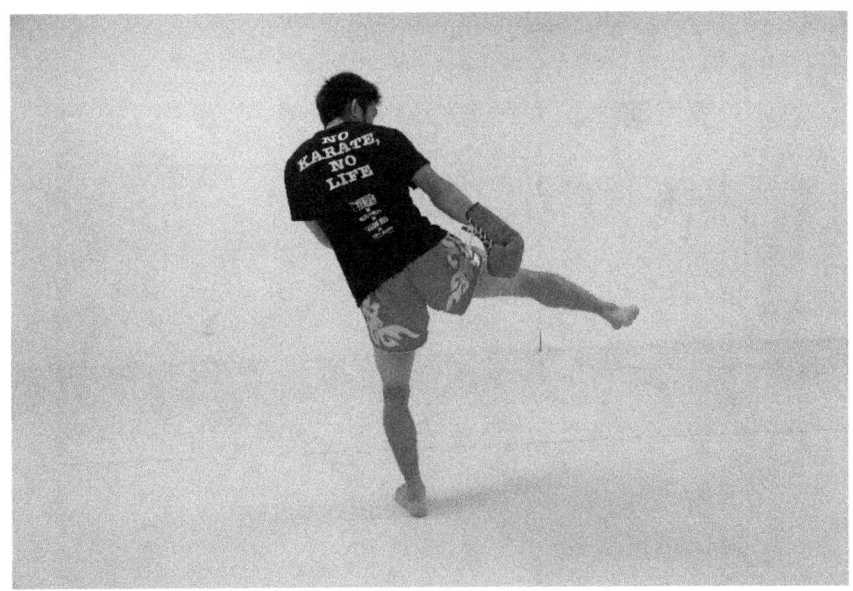

2-10 【Thorax and KO】

Up to this point, it was about the body, mainly about abdomen KO. There is a chest above the abdomen, and the chest is covered with a thorax. The thorax has 12 thoracic vertebrae, 12 pairs of ribs and 1 breast bone jointly formed and is responsible for physical protection and respiration of internal organs .Unlike the abdomen, it is structured like a bird cage made of hard bones, so a different approach than the blows to the abdomen is required. If you strike the thorax with a soft fist you will hurt your hand, so punch and kick to the thorax you can say that some hardness is required. In addition to this, the attack with points becomes extremely effective. When attacking the thorax, stimulation is applied to places with more of the sensation of pain such as the periosteum that wraps the bone as the target part, the ligament around the joint, the soft tissue around it, the intercostal muscle between the ribs, and the pleura behind it, that is going to be the damage to the opponent. The reason why I wrote periosteum surrounding the bone, is because the bone itself has no sensation of pain and the sensation of pain is closely present in the periosteum densely surrounding the bone. The abnormally painful when fracture, is because the periosteum is destroyed.

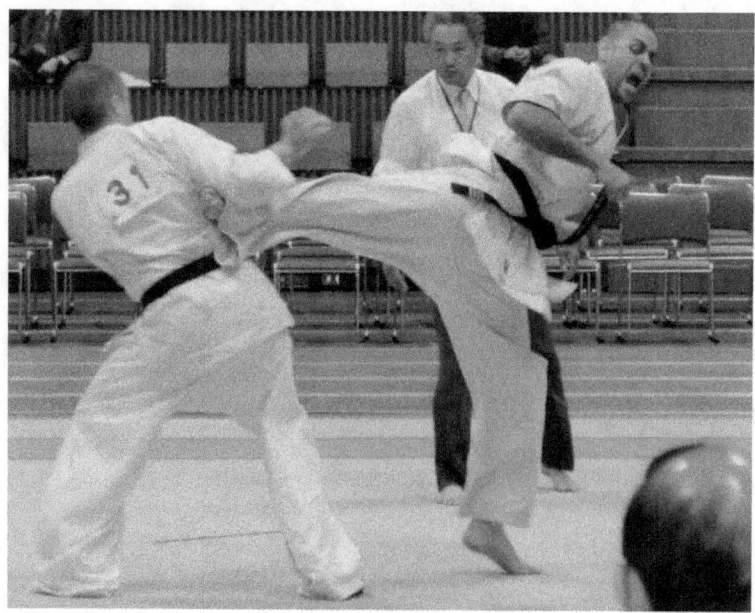

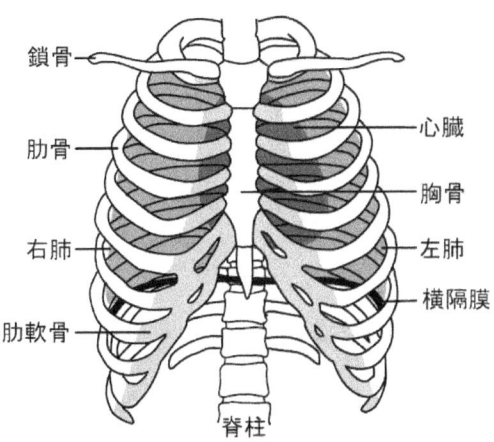

鎖骨 collarbone,clavicle
肋骨 ribs
右肺 pulmo dexter,right lung
肋軟骨 costal cartilage
心臟 heart
胸骨 breastbone,sternum
左肺 left lung,pulmo siniste
横隔膜 diaphragm
脊柱vertebra; spine

In Karate fighting which fought with bare knuckles and feet, the technique of attack on the chest is highly developed, and examples of KO with sternal fracture and rib fracture are also seen. The breastbone has parts such as the manubrium of sternum, corpus sterni, xiphoid process, the part of the joint between the manubrium of sternum and the corpus sterni, and the xiphoid process is a place with many fractures due to external force. Particularly the xiphoid process, because one of them is not connected, so it is structurally easy to break. Likewise for the lower ribs, the spinal column side has a strong connection, but on the opposite side there is no connection between the bones,

69

making it very easy to break. It also feels intolerable pain to get a point blow between ribs.

Do you use fists only in the face or can you take out points at any time? Will you kick the thorax with the face or kick like gnawing the ribs at the foot point? Can you achieve a point hit under wearing an open finger glove? Many striking techniques of "point" such as single fist are seen in Karate and Kenpo before it becomes competitions, and now there are the fighters who revive that in competition as the Japanese expression "visiting old, learn new" are also appearing The pursuit of the blow with point and approach to the thorax may be said to have the possibility of future leap of fighting sports and martial arts.

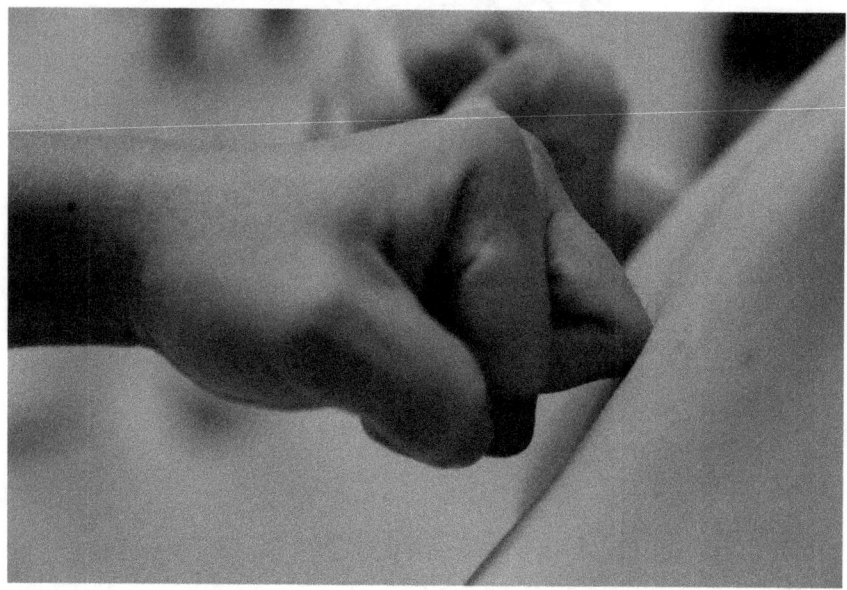

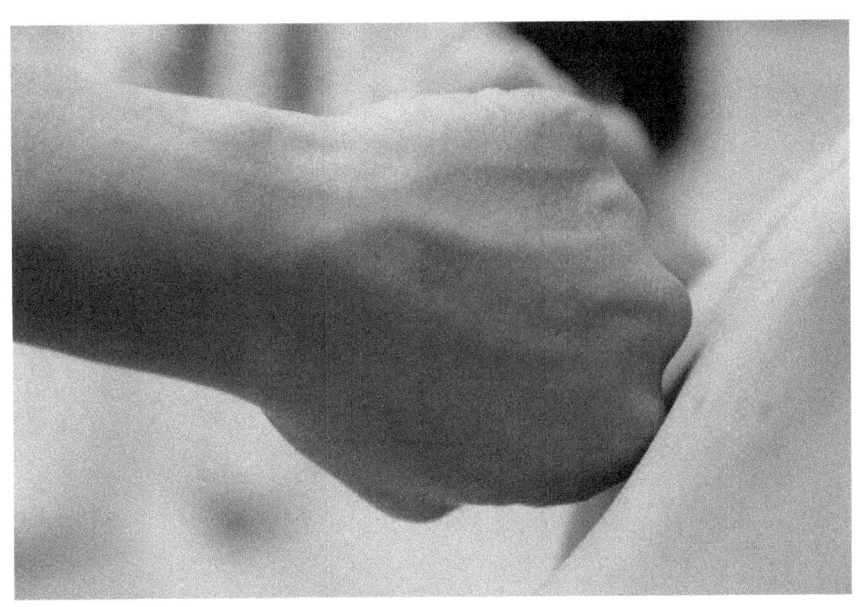

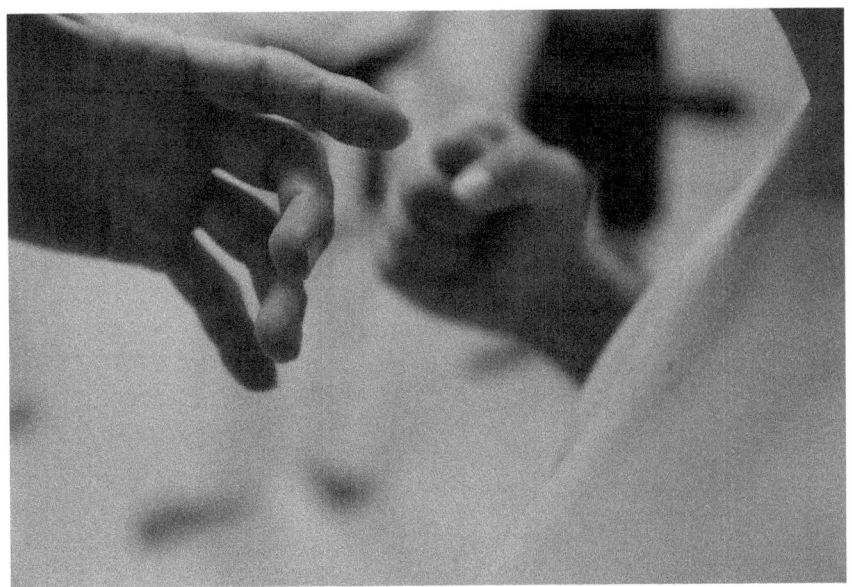

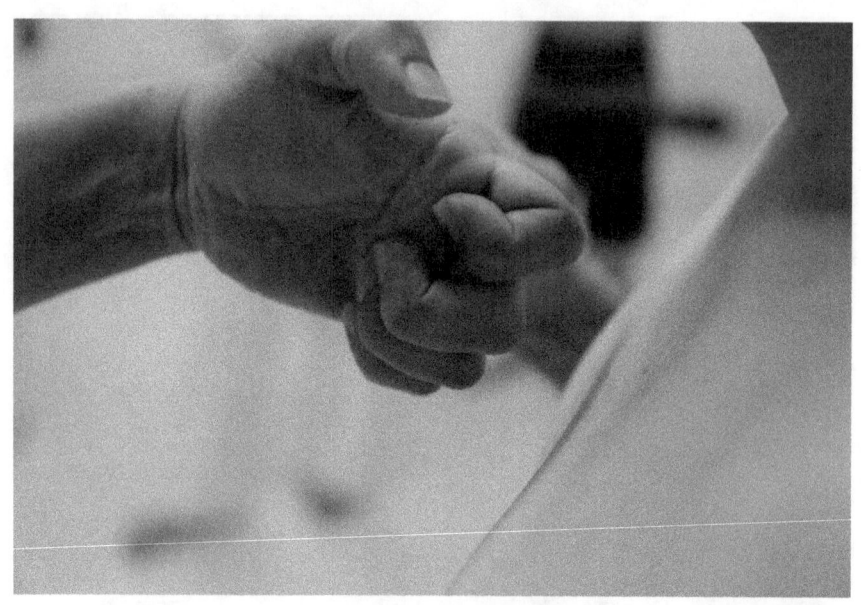

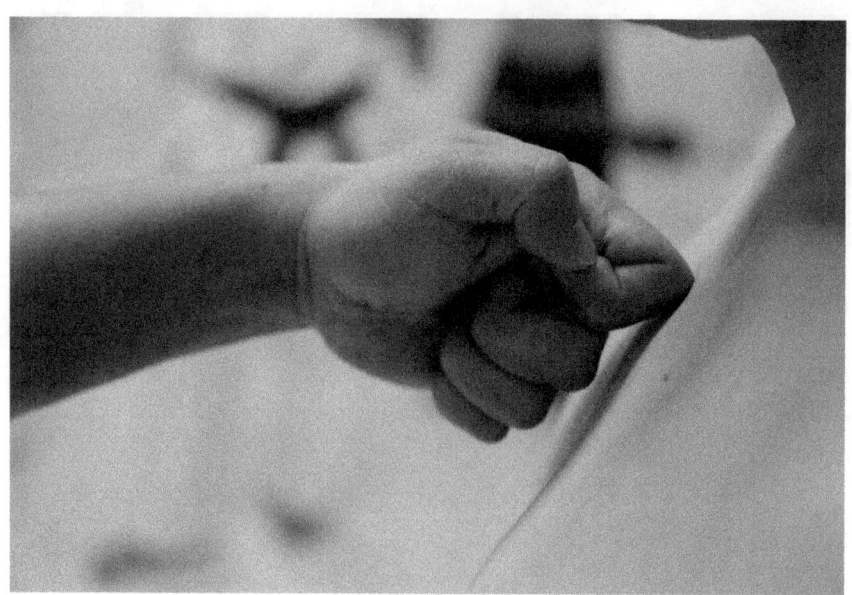

And another thing that I cannot miss is the respiratory function of the thorax. WBA, WBC's former world champion and former Japanese legendary boxer Kuniaki Shibata says He toughly deprived the opponent's stamina with the tactic of keeping his opponent's ribs lightly struck, which was also advantageous against strong foreign fighters. Mr. Eddie who is famous as a great trainer expressed "to break the opponent's tank" to Mr. Shibata. The intercostal muscles between the ribs are deeply involved in breathing as described above, but when the intercostal muscles are subjected to external force, breathing is interrupted. While saying out "ahhhhh", then slap the rib part of your rib cage repeatedly, the sound is cut off as "Ah, ah, ah, ah," the movement of the intercostal muscle is blocked by external force. That is the principle of disturbing breathing. In this case I think that you could understand that the surface is more effective than a point by actually experimenting. Although it does not directly lead to KO, it is one of the tactics to effectively take opponent's stamina and increase the opportunity of KO.

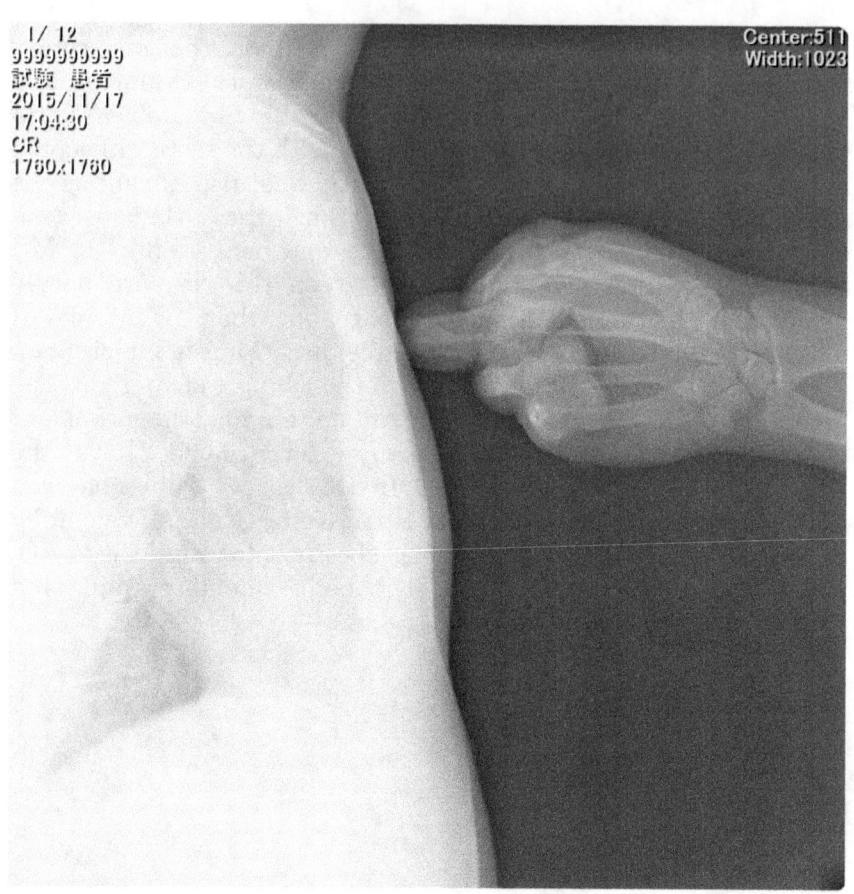

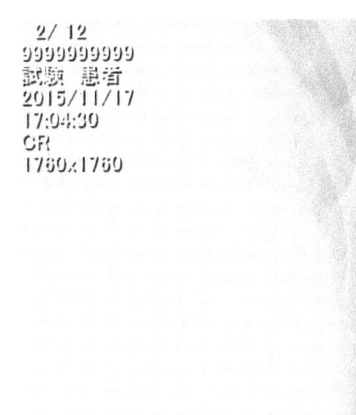

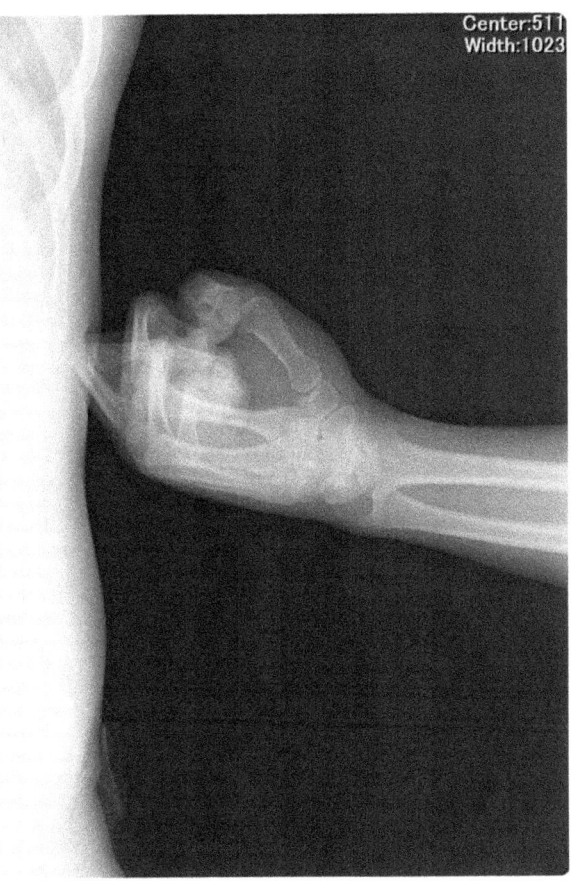

2-11 【Technics and tactics】

By knowing more deeply and accurately the structure of the body and thorax, the barrier function of the abdominal muscles, the relationship with the respiration, technology and tactics may evolve greatly. Even when you punch on the body, if you strike against the opponent whom is firmly stood, the barrier of your opponent's abdominal muscle becomes very effective. If you use other techniques or feints to destabilize your opponent's balance, the moment of collapse will give priority to contraction to the muscle group to restore the stability to stabilize, so the barrier function will decline. If you move thinking about not having "opponent's right straight" or not taking it, the opportunities for attacks like a sharp gnawing point strike to the right rib will also gets to be zero, at the moment of the opponent's right straight. The stronger the right straight of the opponent, the greater the damage to the opponent due to the synergistic effect. I think it's wasteful not to use it. Even though the form of the technique is the same, the influence on the opponent greatly depends on "when to put out", "which timing to put out" and "creating what kind of situation to put out". Creating skills by understanding humans, and make effort to improve them to be able to construct the technics and tactics with confidence, is the interesting aspect of the scientific and medical point of view.

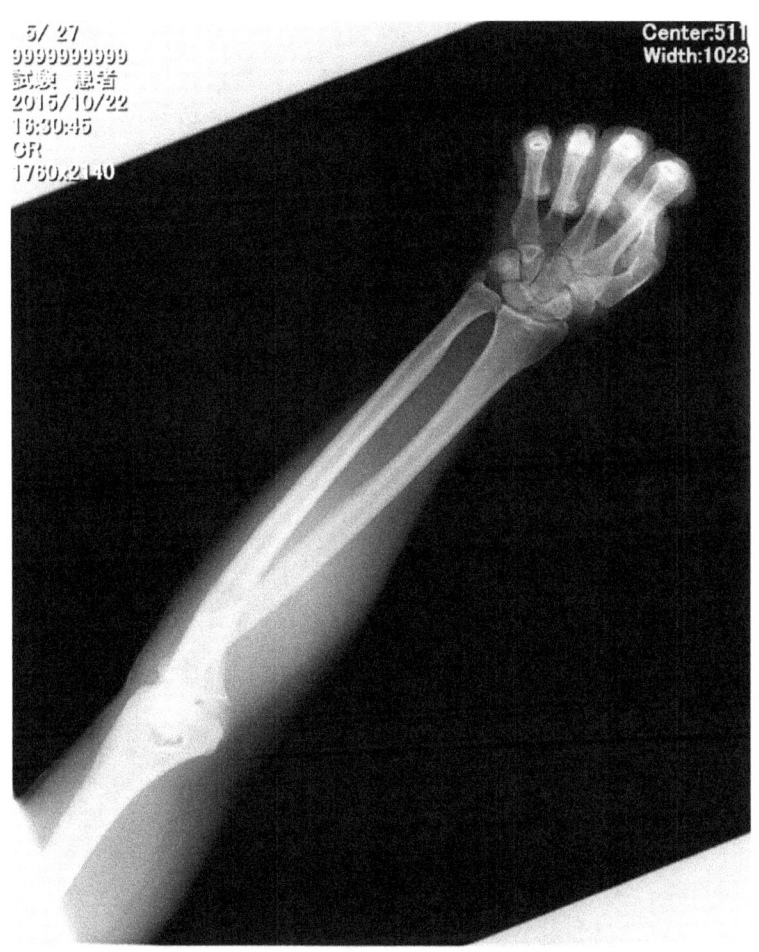

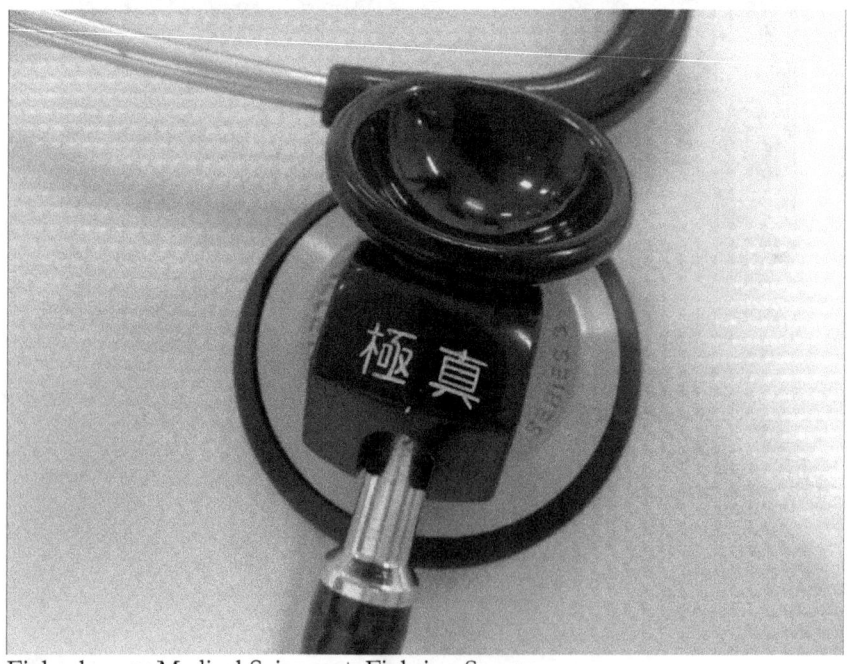

Fightology = Medical Science + Fighting Sports
Please find you own answer and create your style.

3:What Is KO?
-Low Kick-

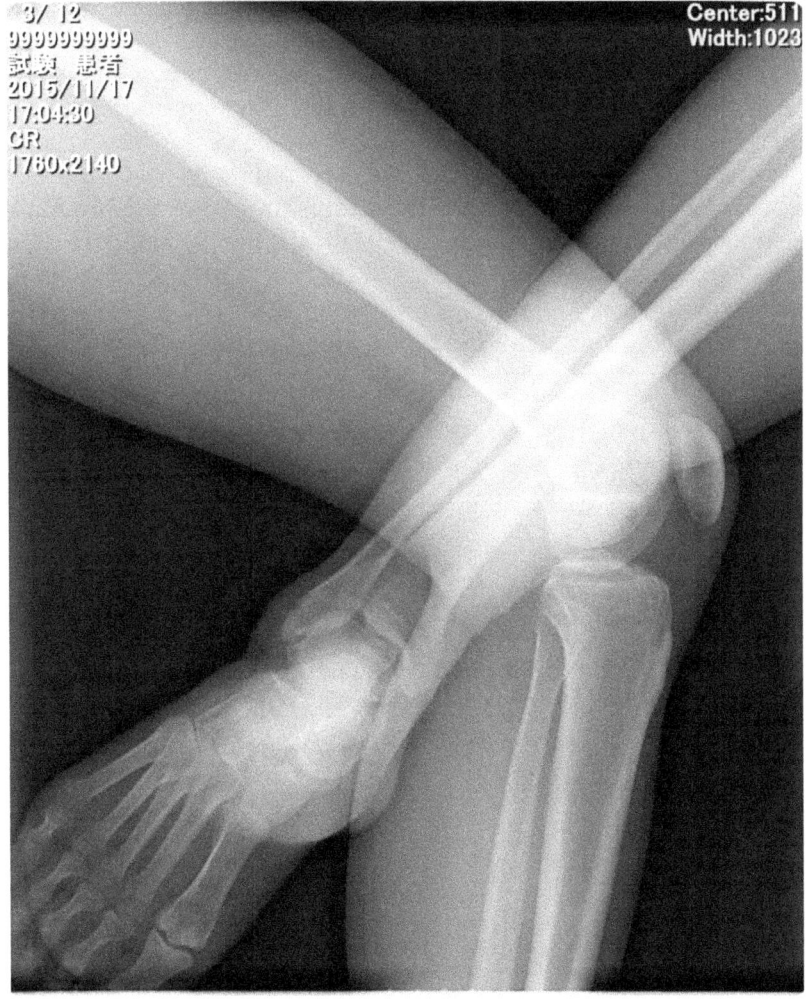

3-1 【KO with low kick】

Gedan-geri, low kick.

With a kicking technique that deals great damage if you take it accurately, the kick of a skilled low kicker is the destructive power reminiscent of "fine Japanese sword". It is unbearable painful technic that only practitioners can know, which is unknown to those who have never kicked like that. The variation of low kick is steadily increasing, and one of the technics that is still evolving. Actually there is a case that the thigh bone which is the thickest bone in the human body has gotten broken by a low kick during the match and it is a kick technique to lose the opponent's "hope" sometimes, contrary to the simple look from the outside .

The principles were that the KO system on the face is about "rotating the brain rapidly due to external force (technique) to cause concussion", abdominal KO system "to release the protecting function of abdominal muscle to stimulate peritoneal pain sense which causes pain. So, in the case of the lower attacks, how is KO created by kicking against the opponent's lower limb, such as gedan-geri or lower kick? Let's consider the mechanism from an anatomical point of view.

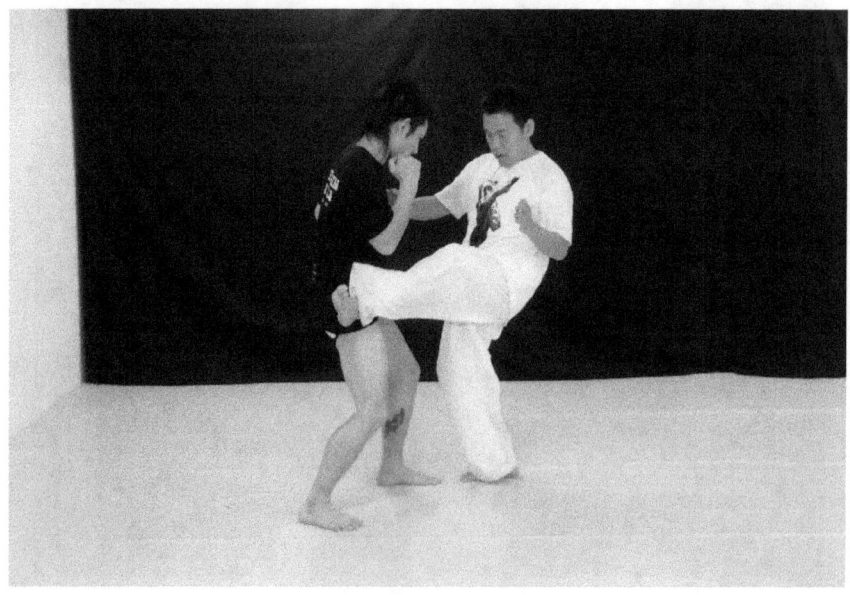

3-2 【Experiment】

Let's make a pair and let the partner kick your buttocks. At first, please get kicked lightly and gradually make it stronger. I think it will hurt with the increased power of kicking, If you have some level of martial art experience, you will not get enough damage that makes you can't move even if you get a bit strong kick.

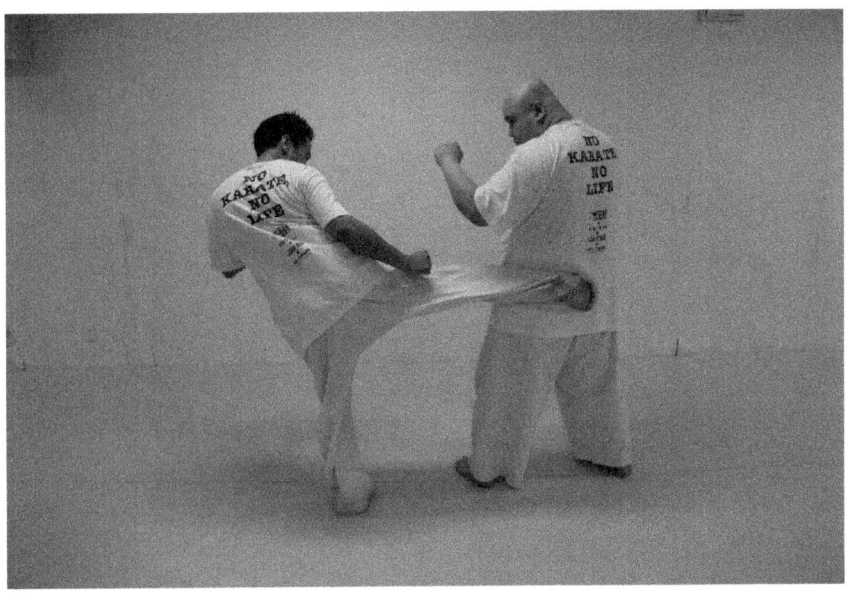

Up to some generations ago in Japan, there used to be a "Slapping buttocks" skill? had been practiced commonly to punish a naughty kid. It's not a proper way if it is an abuse only, or if the parents have the notion of only for distracting their emotion, but there are people whom did it or being done based on their care, and the message is passed on to the kid, as well as hoping the kid knows the pain itself for his/her experience. Aside from the argument of 'abuse' or 'upbringing', from the perspective of Society of fighting medicine's, if we consider it as a strike, "Slapping buttocks" enters a category of high safety. The buttocks cover the hip joints that are used repeatedly in everyday life such as standing up and sitting down, walking and running, and large and thick muscle groups such as the gluteus maximus and subcutaneous tissue cover like a protector, so that this is the part relatively strong to the external force.

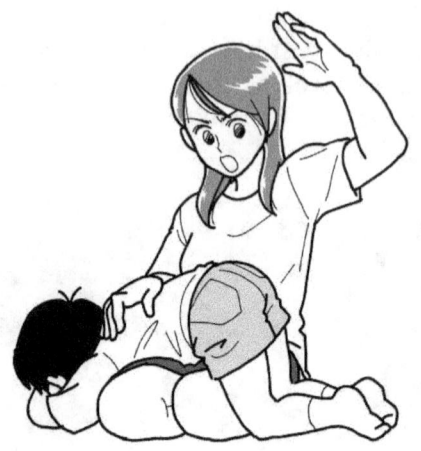

The founder of Kyokushin Karate, Mr. Masutatsu Oyama, when he was in training, when he was unable to demonstrate his strength during training to lift a high weight barbell, he was telling his wife "to stab his buttocks with a futon needle(which is relatively thick and long compared to the other sewing needles)". In order to demonstrate intense power, the original methodology that seems extreme case was consideration of safety which leads to the aftereffect with low possibility.

The head of a child whose brain grows day by day, there are almost no gaps, so intracranial bleeding and the like tend to cause cerebral herniation, which is a very high risk of losing the life. Because the chest, back, upper abdomen are close to the heart, the risk of Cardiac Concussion which is prone to children is increased. Cardiac Concussion is also a part to be avoided absolutely because the mortality rate is extremely high. Knee joints, shoulder joints, etc. are also at high risk of ligament injury, fracture and dislocation, and there is also the possibility of functional impairment. Unrepairable parts such as eyes and lower abdomen are extremely dangerous even for adults, and there is a high possibility of leaving aftereffects. Looking at each part like this, I think that "Slapping buttocks" is a safe wisdom as a pain stimulation to a part where functional impairment is hard to bear, with a very little risk of life-related damage. Of course, it is better to say and tell the story, I am not really recommending you to do "Slapping buttocks" "Receiving a gedan-geri or a low kick in the buttocks" is an effective choice of avoiding a KO. Some fighter uses a technic using the buttock to receive the strike when he/she really can't avoid a hit. Through this experiment, I think you can now realize that KO is hard to do (to be done by) at the part covered with thick muscle groups.

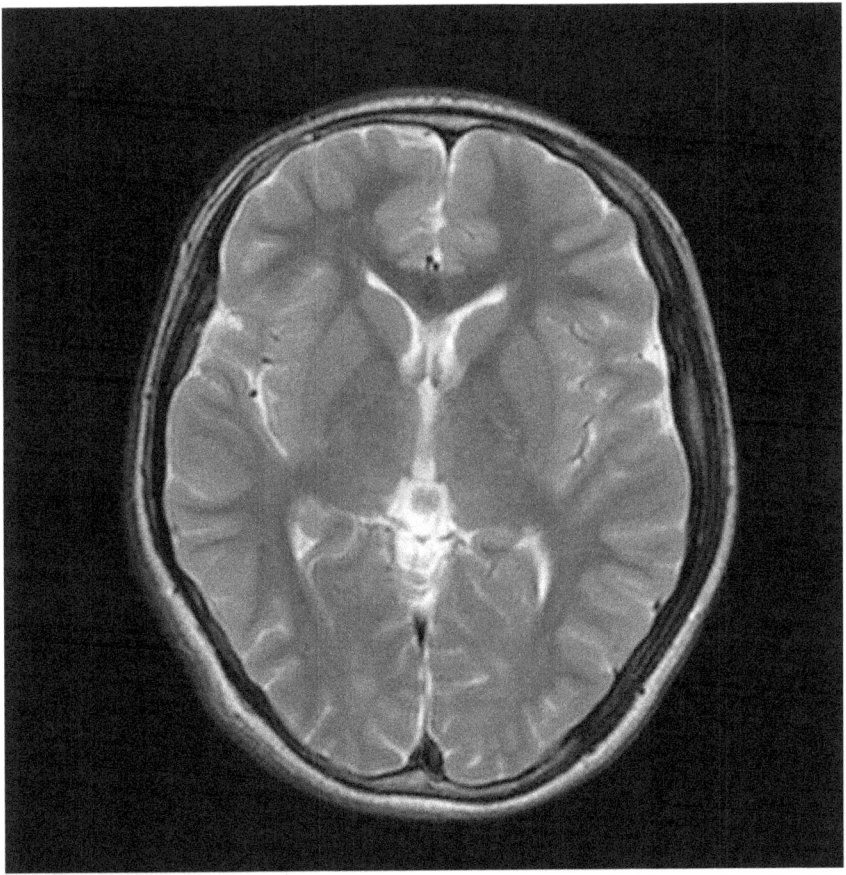

(Brain CT of teenager.)

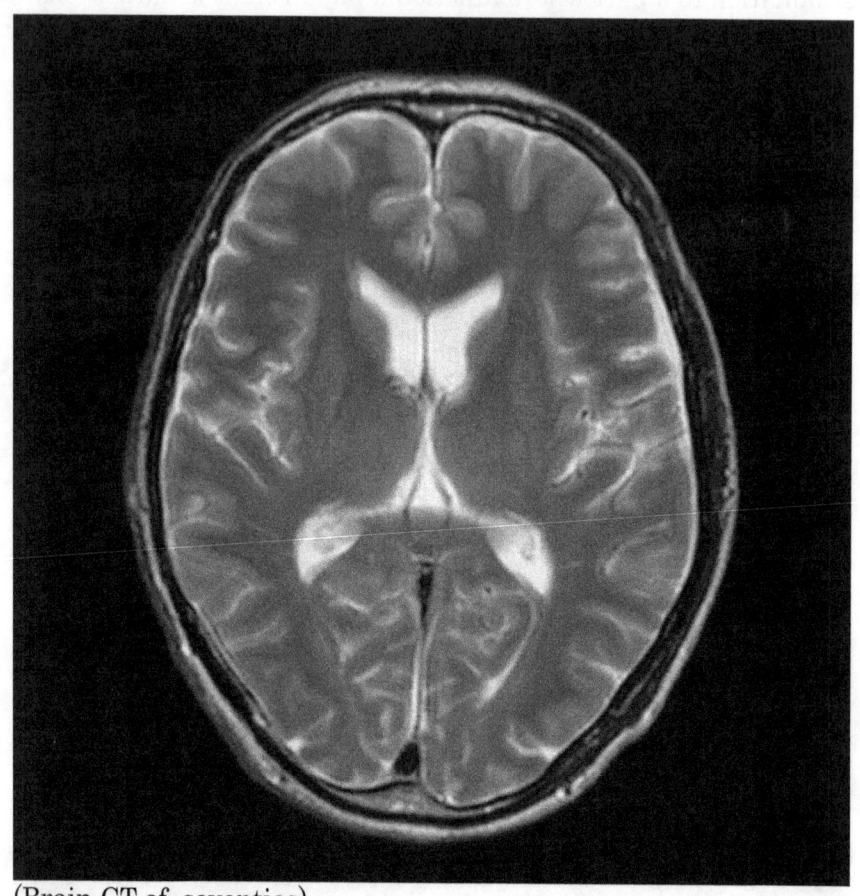

(Brain CT of seventies)

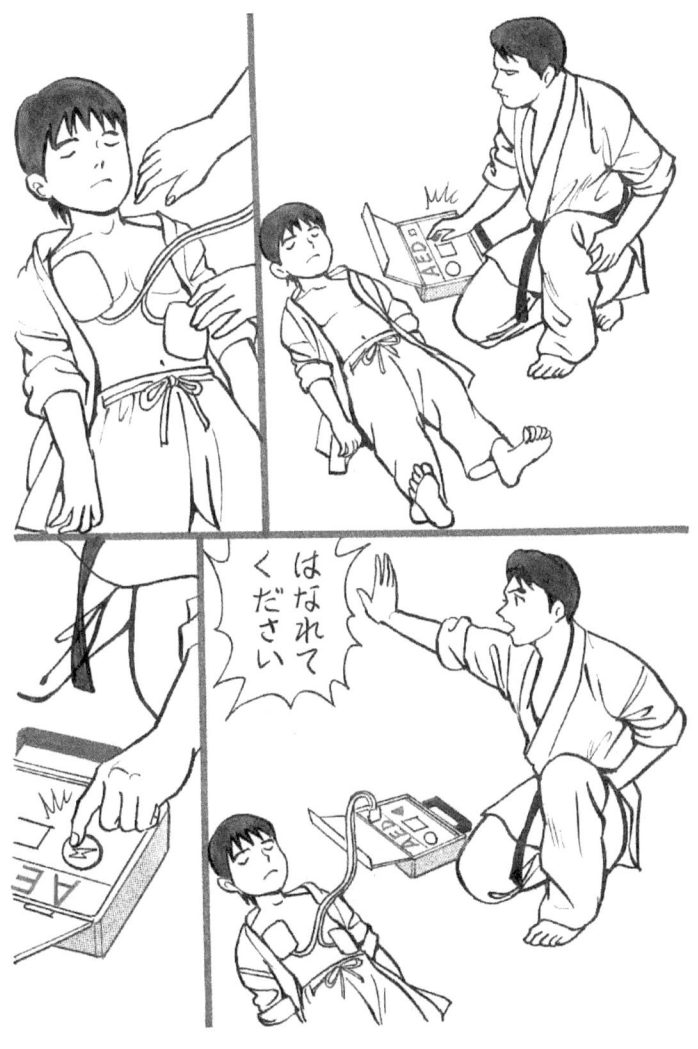

(Cardiac Concussion →AED)

3-3 【Lower limb anatomy】

Here, let me explain the anatomy of the lower limb. Lower limbs are grown from the pelvis. The femur (thigh bone) forms a hip joint so as to be in contact with the part of the pelvic side called the acetabulum. Looking at the image of CT, the lower limbs from the hip joint come out rearward and downward and outward. If you touch the outside of the hip joint, I think you may touch a hard part just under the skin, but call that part, greater trochanter. In the femur, the greater trochanter is on the outside and behind. From there, the femur extends inward and forward. And as you approach the knee, it will move to the front of the thigh. When taking a posture of "At attention" and closing the toes, when looking at the right lower limb only from right in front, the lower part of the "L" shape is longer form. Viewed from the outside (right side), the lower part of the "L" shape is also positioned longer. Until I myself studied anatomy properly, I only had the image of the thigh bone is growing straight in the middle of the thigh. Actually, I was not running in the middle, and it was showing the "L" shape. As a result of shooting again CT scan, we were able to confirm again that the structure of the femur is closely linked to the KO by the low kicks.

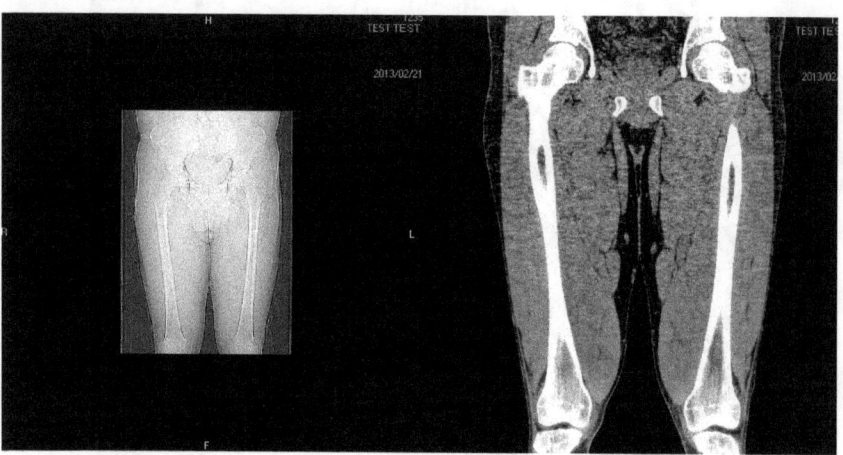

3-4 【Area with much sensation of pain】

Humans have sensation of pain. Sensation of pain is a sensory receptor that senses pain as it says, but pain receptor is present in the body and constantly sends its information to the center. The more pain receptors are, the more pain is felt, the less painful the place where the number is small. The ear lobe that pierce the earring is a part where the number of pain receptors is relatively small, and there are so many pain receptors such as in the eyeballs. Even with the hand, on the palm side and on the back of the hand, the pain that you feel with the same stimulation, they are totally different. Since the part with a lot of receptors is a part deeply related to the maintenance and function of the living body, it is also a high priority part that must be protected. Always a lot of sensors are watching and even small damage will be informed to the brain as soon as a painful stimulation happens.

Pain receptors are also distributed densely in the joints and their surroundings. The muscles become tendons via the muscle-tendon junction, and the tendons adhere to the periosteum. Muscle-tendon junction is a part whose property changes with muscle and tendon, one part which is prone to rupture when load concentrates. There are a lot of pain receptors on the muscle-tendon junction and tendon because it hinders moving the body where the tendons rupture. Like the rib cage, there are no pain receptors in the bones themselves even in the lower limbs. Receptors of the sensation of pain are dense in the periosteum which wraps the bone itself. The unique "unbearable pain" that fracture gives is not a bone itself but a pain stimulation on pain receptors of the periosteum. Ligament is an important tissue linking joints to joints, and because it breaks down function of the joint itself when rupturing, it is the tissue which is rich in pain receptors. Joint techniques such as leg lock and upper cross arm lock are external forces on tendons and ligaments that tend to feel pain.

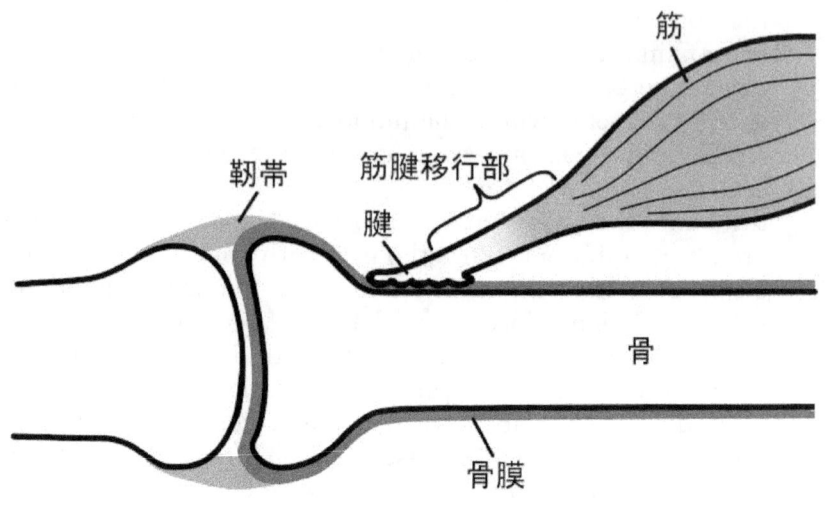

筋 muscle
筋腱移行部 muscle-tendon junction, musculotendinous transition
腱 tendon
靭帯 ligament
骨 bone
骨膜 periosteum

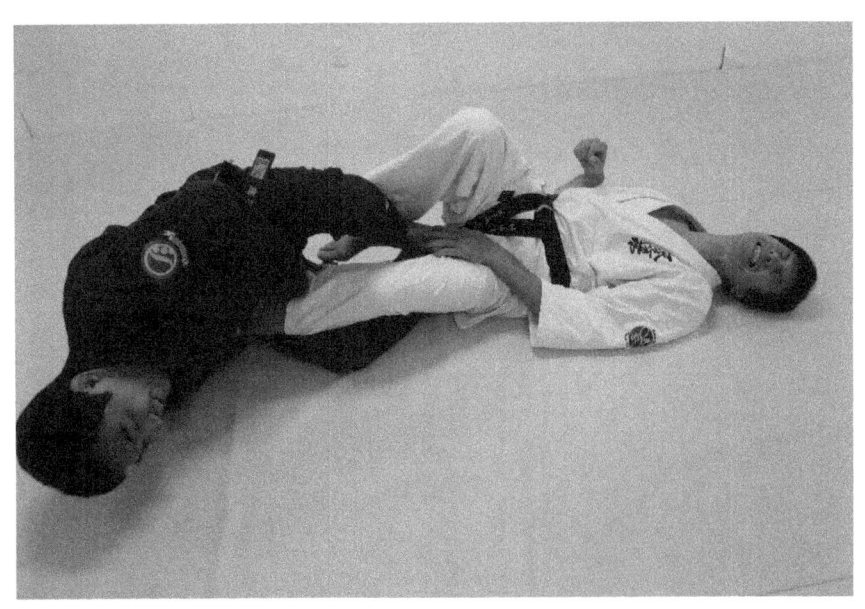

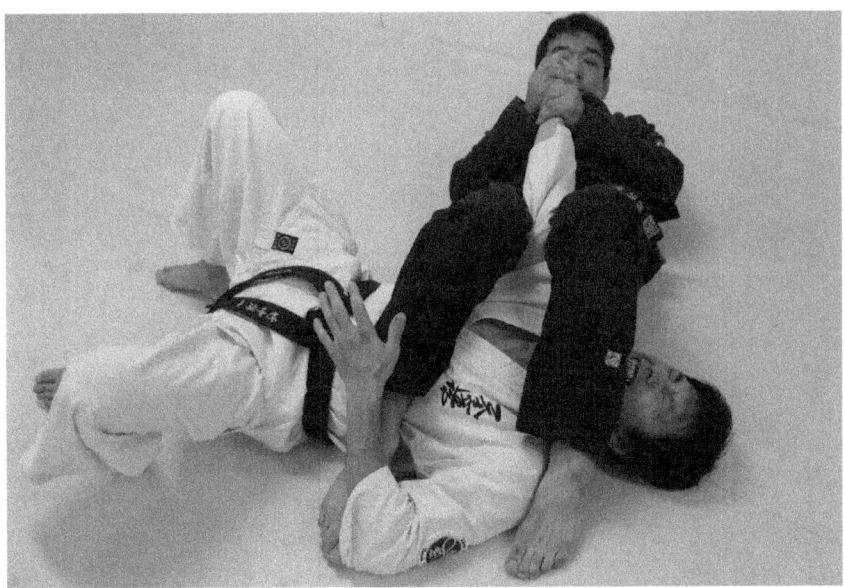

3-5 【Points that collapse by low kick and damage on the kicking side】

When targeting the lower limb with a low kick or a gedan-geri,

(A) Muscle and other protectors are thin
(B) a site with many pain receptors,

It is a shortcut to KO to aim at. For the identification of that part, it is very useful to run the bones with the CT images mentioned above.

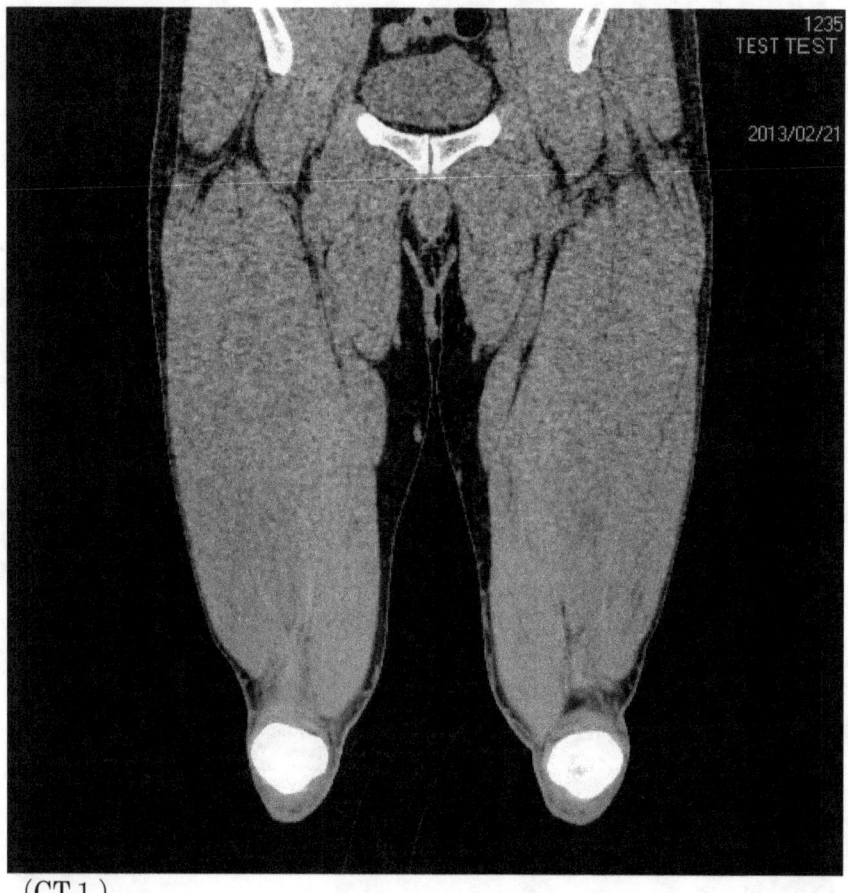

(CT 1)

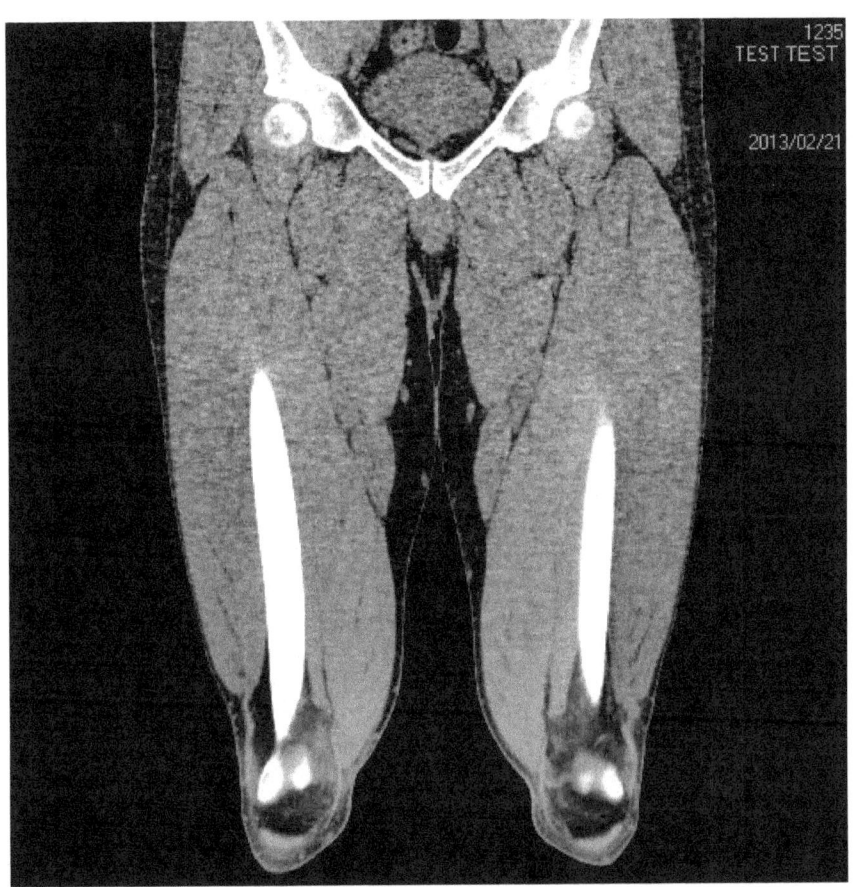

（CT2）

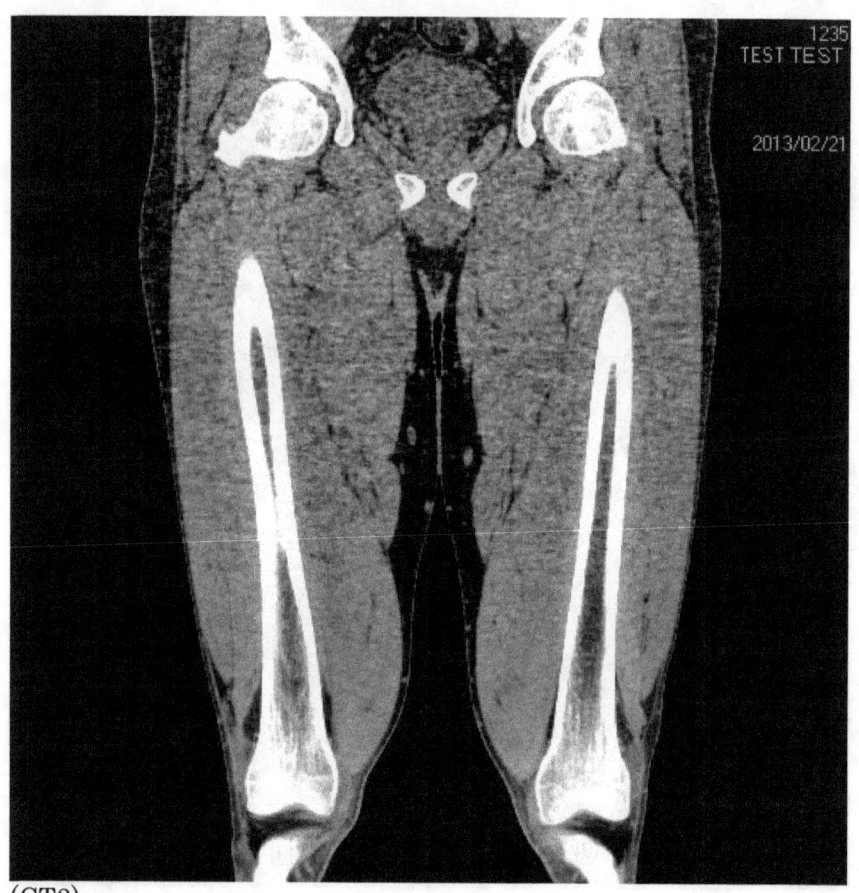

(CT3)

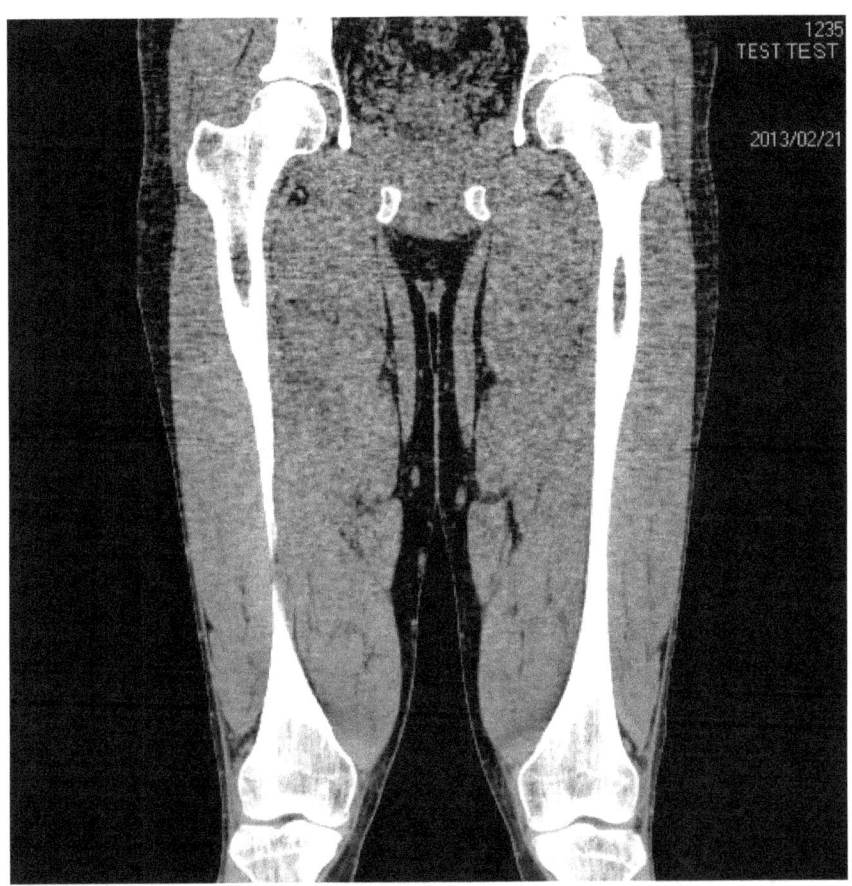

(CT4)

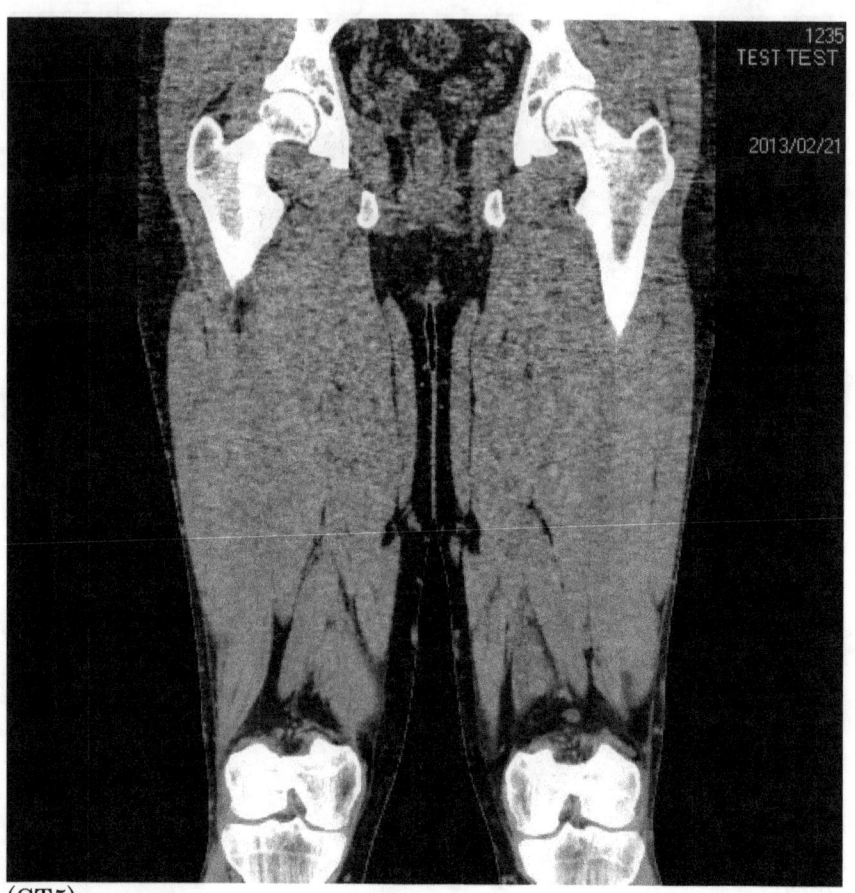

(CT5)

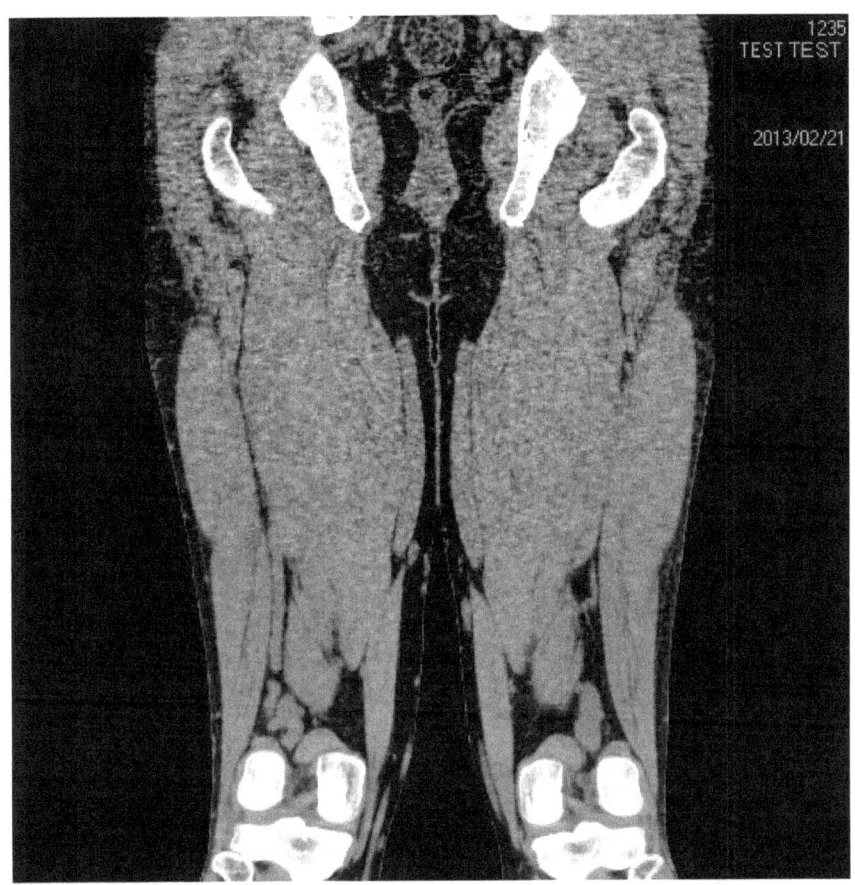

(CT6)

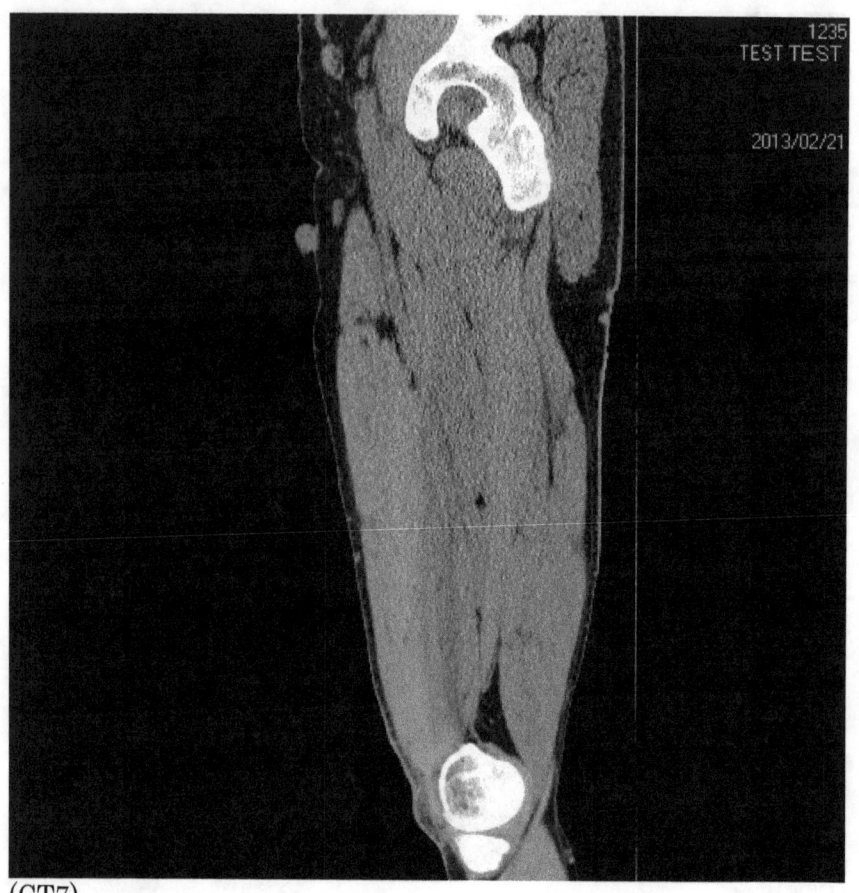

(CT7)

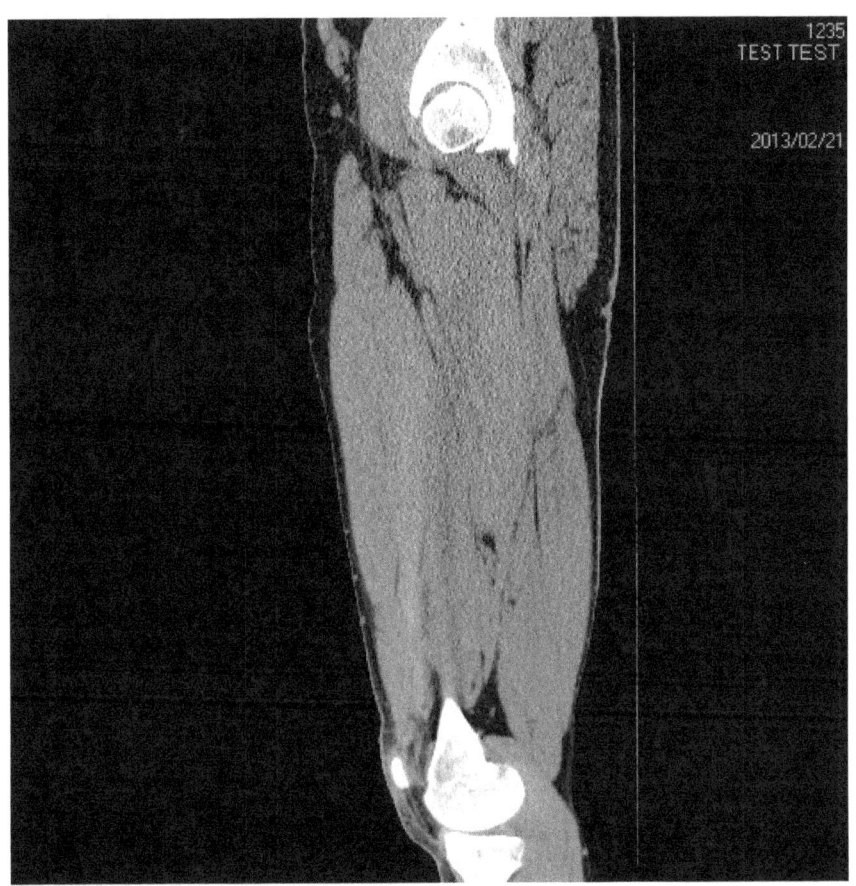

(CT8)

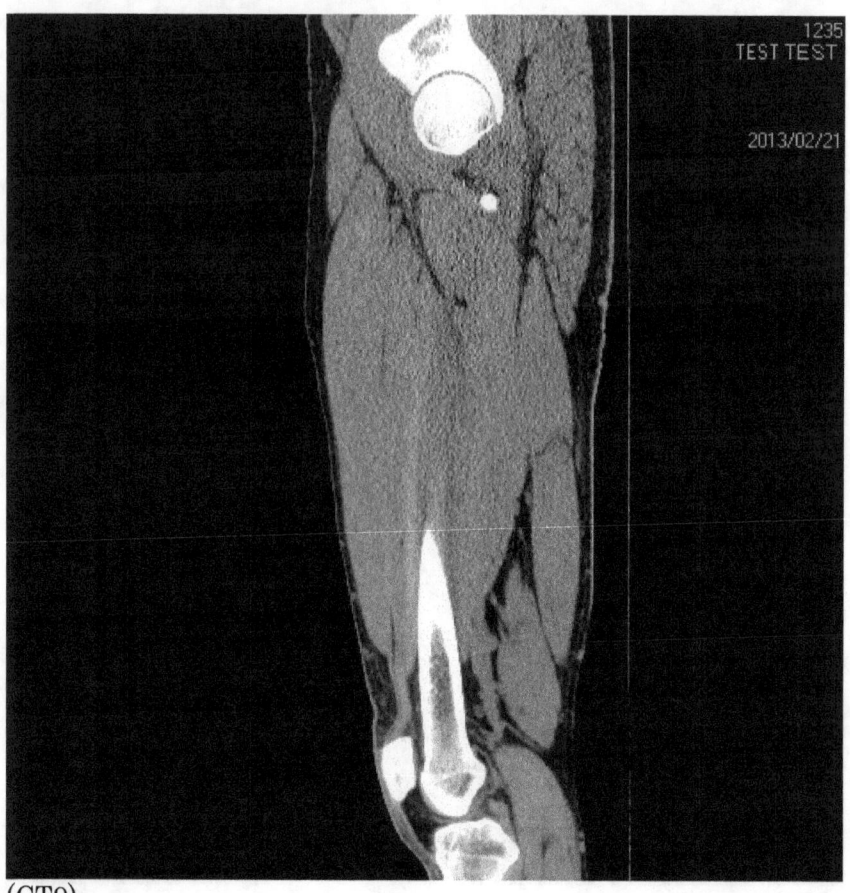

(CT9)

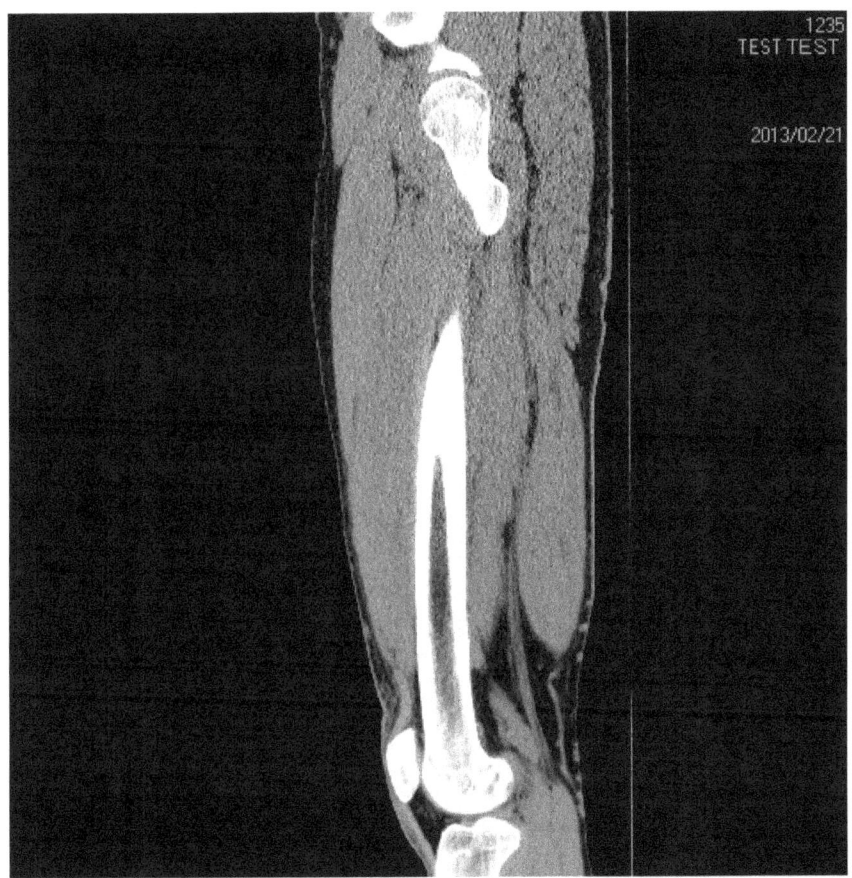

(CT10)

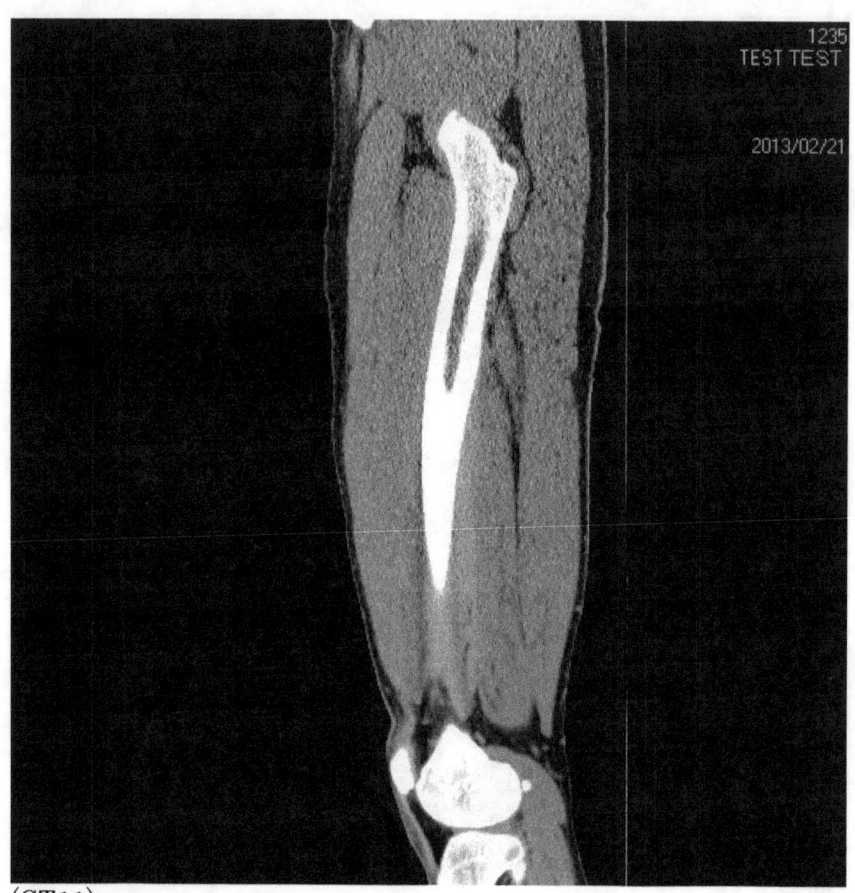

(CT11)

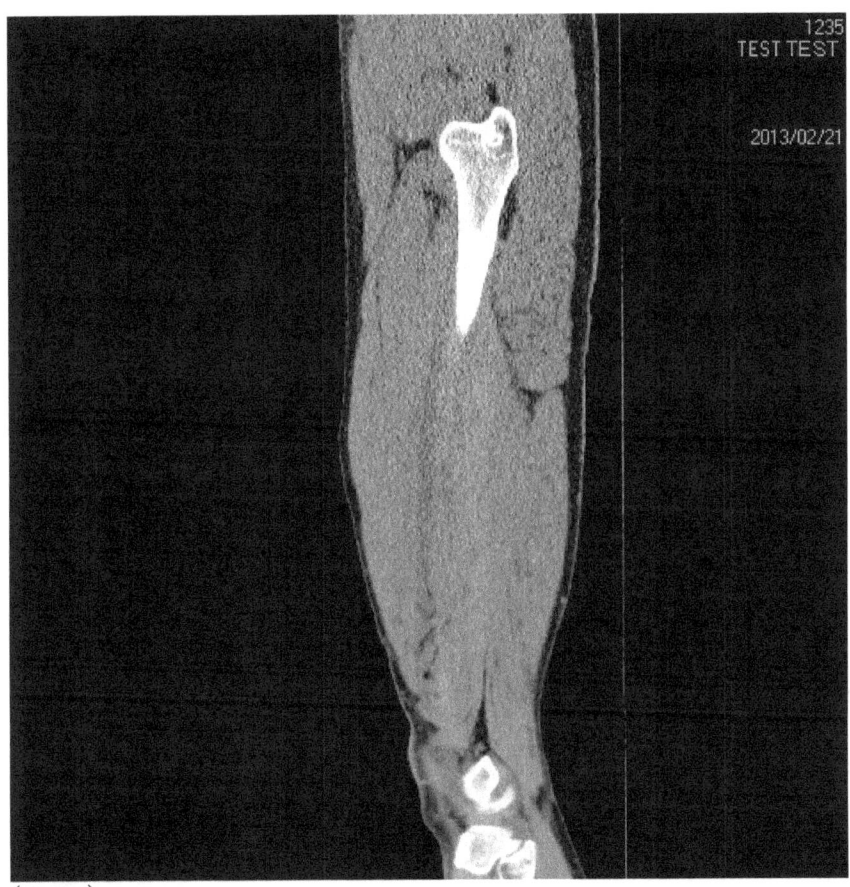

(CT12)

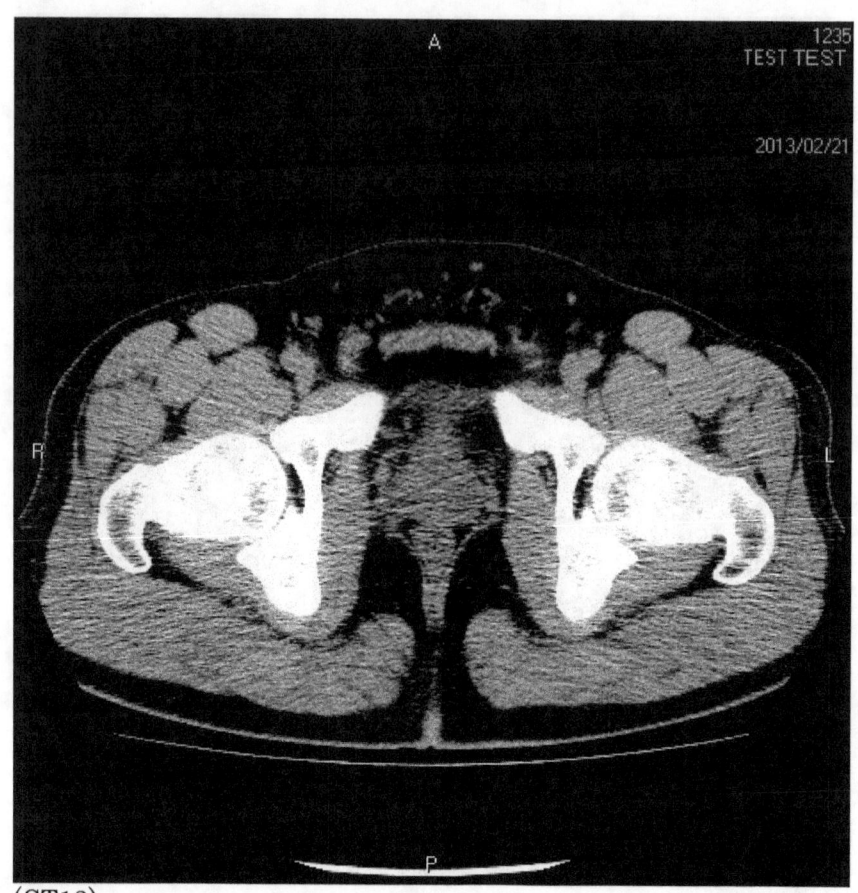

(CT13)

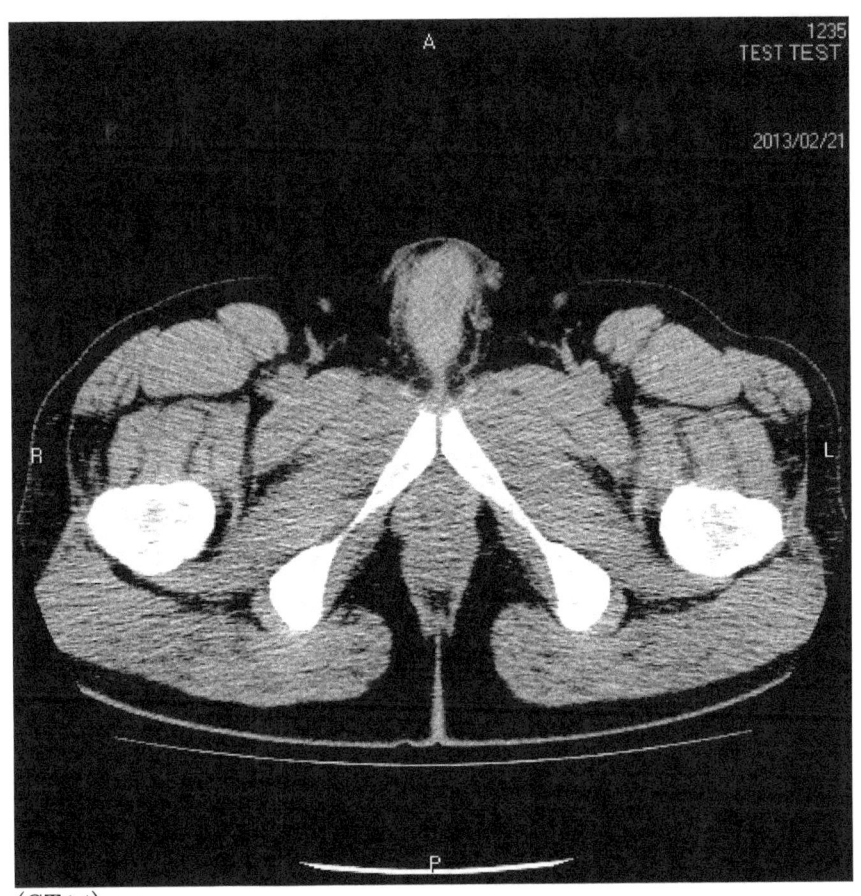

(CT14)

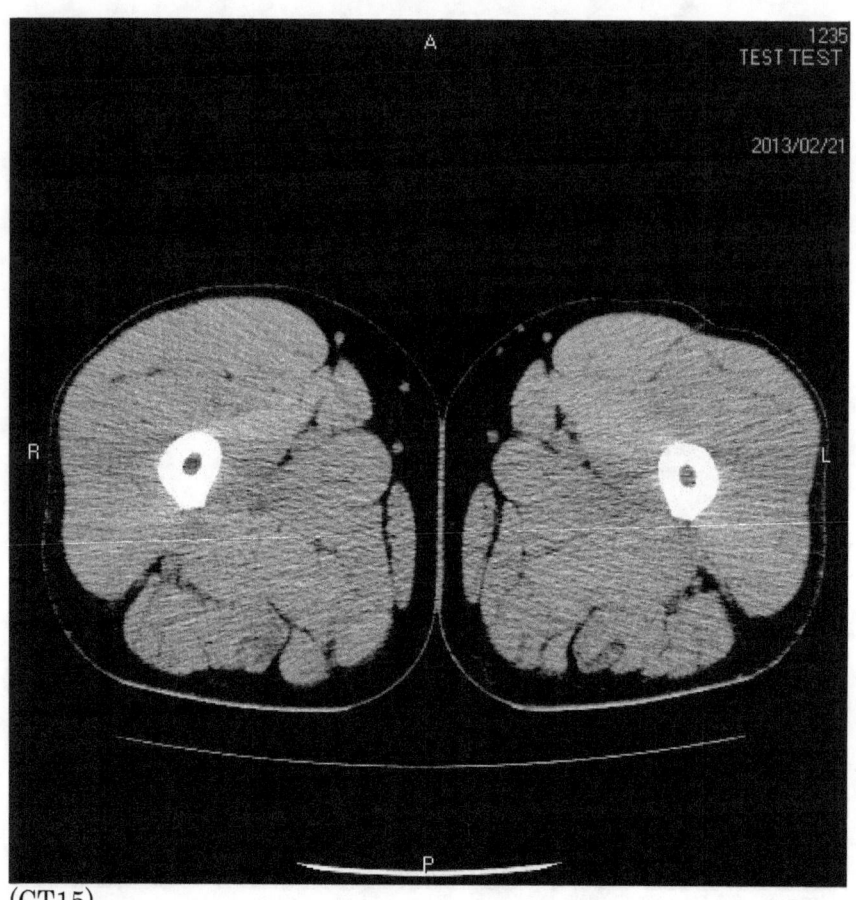

(CT15)

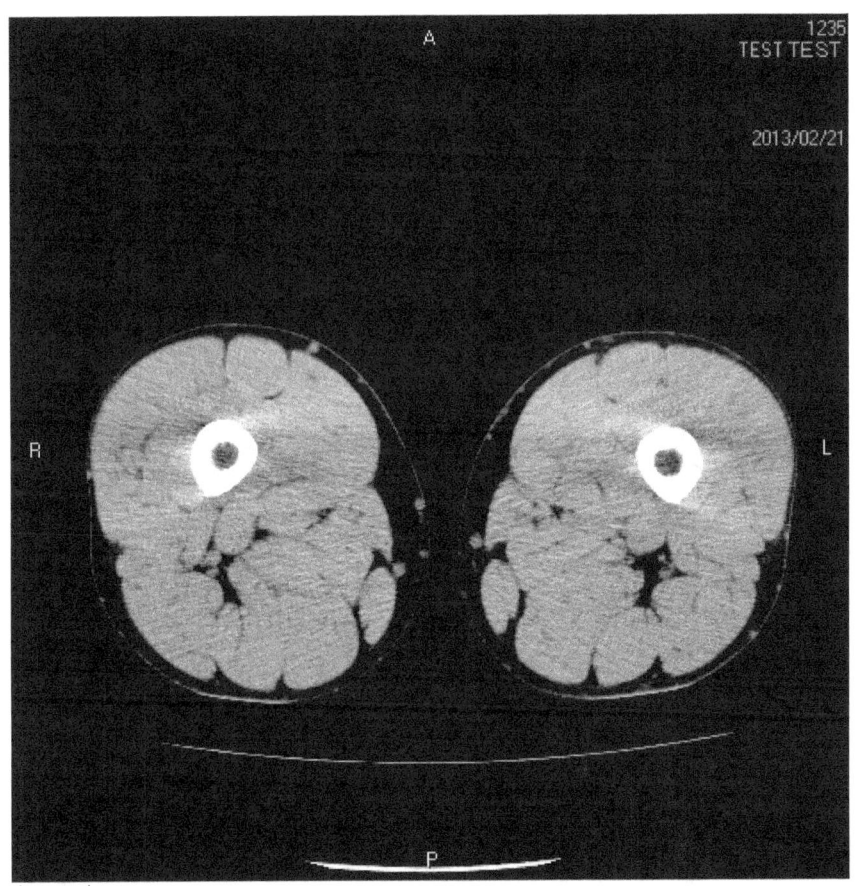

(CT16)

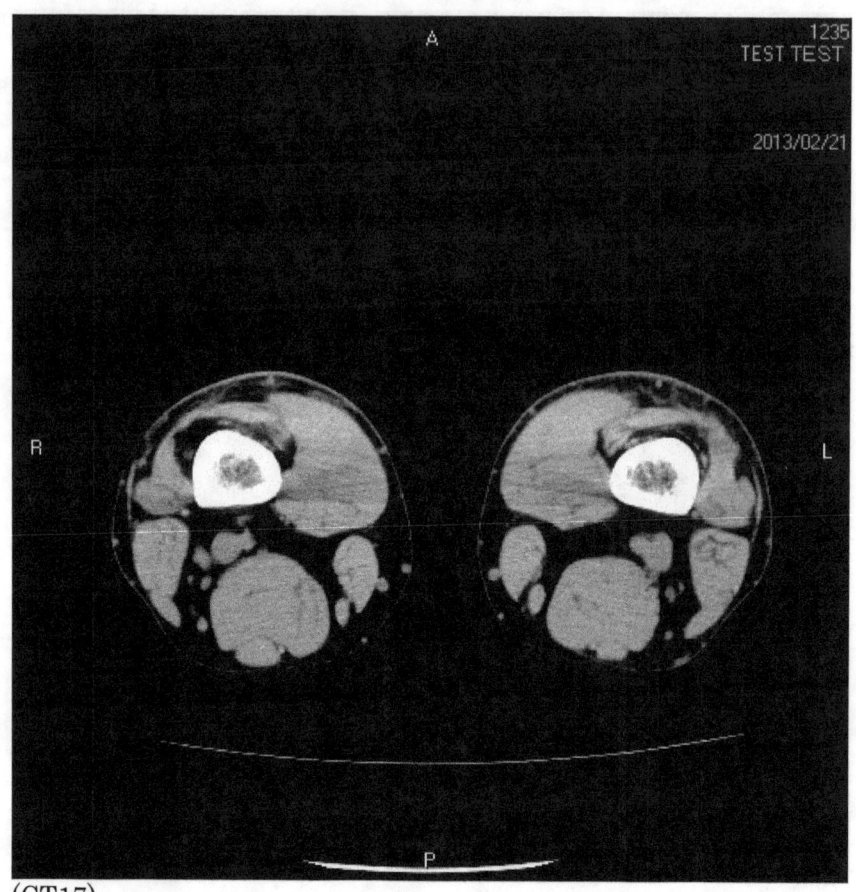

(CT17)

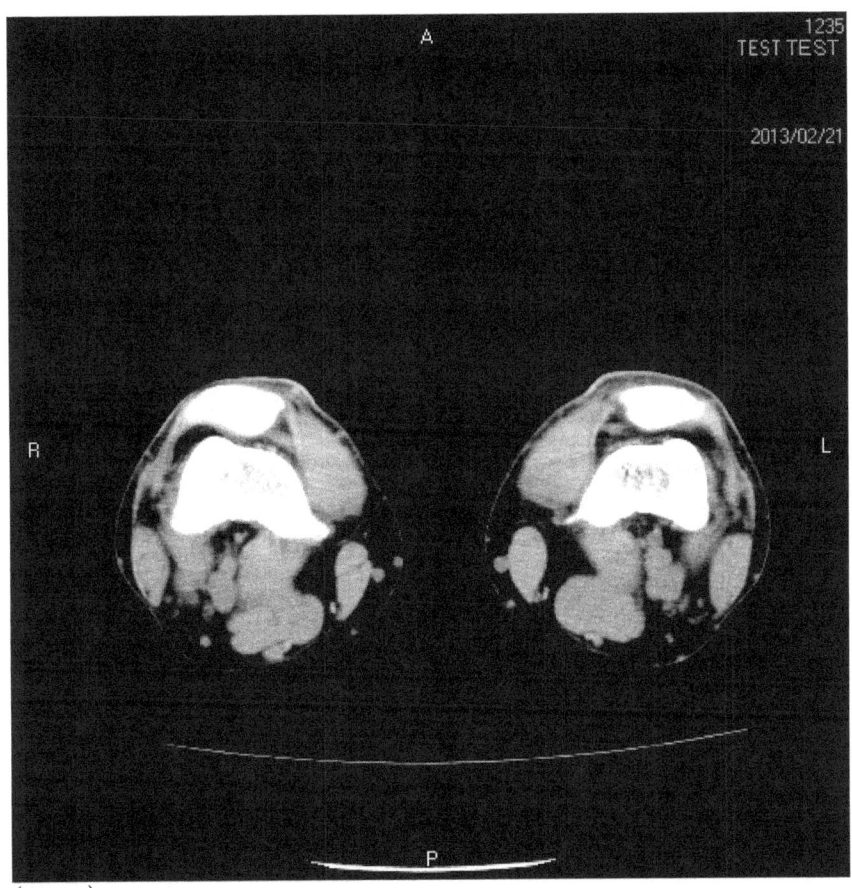

(CT18)

CT images 1 to 6 are parallel to the forehead, sliced from the front of the body, front to back. 1 is front (abdomen side), 6 is back (back side). The closer the knee is, the femur is in front, the closer it is to the hip joint, the more thigh bone is located behind, you may be able to observe from the images. The subsequent CT images 7 to 12 are sliced in the vertical direction and are located from the inside of the thigh to the outside. (7 is inside, 12 is outside). The part near the knee is located inside, the big trochanter near the hip joint is located outside. And 13 to 18 slice horizontally from the pelvis to the knee, is from the top to the bottom. The greater trochanter is located outside the hip joint and slightly backwards, then the thighbone is shifted front side and inward. Looking from a position close to the height of the pelvis in three dimensions that is liable to collapse by the low kick based on these CT images, the surroundings of the hip joint, the greater trochanter located somewhat behind the hip joint, the right front of the thigh bone near the knee, the medial collateral ligament and the radial collateral ligament of the knee joints could be said to be a representative part satisfying both AB conditions. If you are kicking the thigh from the front, the part closer to the knee is more effective. If you are kicking a low kick to the inner thigh, it is more effective at a position lower than the high position of the thigh. Anatomically grasping "running of bone" and giving a physical stimulation such that a part rich in pain receptors is pinched between your bone and the opponent's bone. This is the mechanism of the occurrence of pain in the low kicks.

Gaining hard power and speed, kick it without hesitation on anywhere! The opponent will collapse if you hit it! The way you hold an image like that is also necessary, but in the low kick, the more you kick, the more your feet, the more ligature you will bear the burden. Unlike the case of kicking the face and body, the target is the physically strong lower body which supports the opponent's weight, so low kicks and gedan-geris are also "double edged sword" due to the nature of the technique. In a heavy opponent or a durable opponent, in the continuous fights in a harsh tournament, the damage which the kicked side accumulates becomes larger. While pursuing power and speed, the pursuit of precision with the theme "Which point do you want to match with which point of the opponent" is not only leading to increased damage to the opponent, but also in the harsh battle, it will also reduce your own damage.

3-6 【Adjust point to point】

Let's pair up for two people and look for the aim point of the low kick. Let's search for rich parts of sensation of pain with knock knock to search pinpoint with a grip way called Naka-Daka -Ipponken (a karate fist grip which you hold the fist with the middle finger's second joint as prominent part to hit). If there is a part that is more stimulating than the surroundings, stimulated with the same strength, that part is a weak point. Learn that weak point firmly and try to make it possible for you to reproduce immediately with your body as well. Next step is to explore where to hit my kicks. The proximal part of the first metatarsal bone of the foot, the tibia which is the shin bone, the calcaneus when the heel kicking, etc. are stimulated similarly with the knock knock sound.

Human body is interesting, if stimulation is applied at a point, it becomes easy to be conscious of points to be called a strong point. Normally, consciousness becomes more rough because be conscious on one point of lower limbs separately and the information becomes too much and it cannot be processed. If you kick roughly, you are likely to become a kick that kicks the surface with the surface by all means, so in order to have consciousness of the point, please also try "An effort" to make good use of physical stimulation . And please try to find the point where you can conquer your opponent enoughly with a little force.

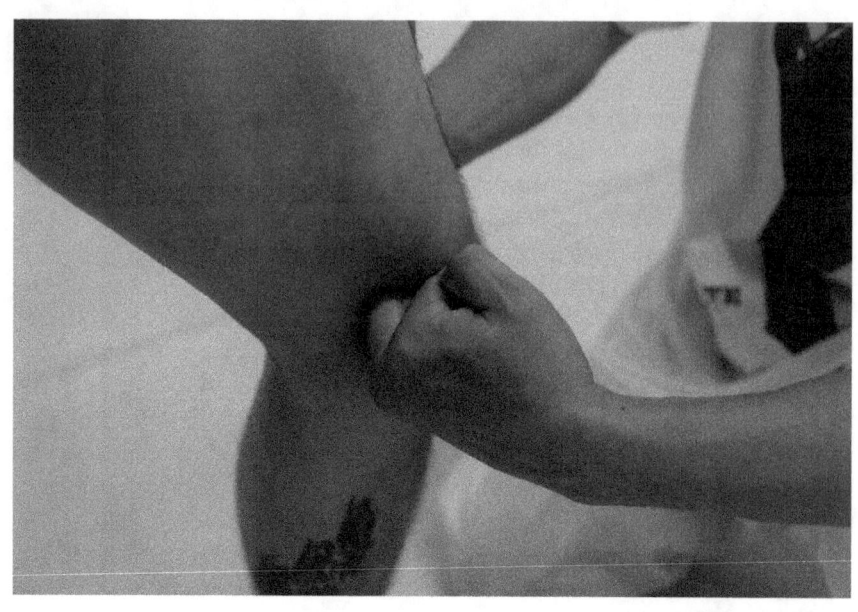

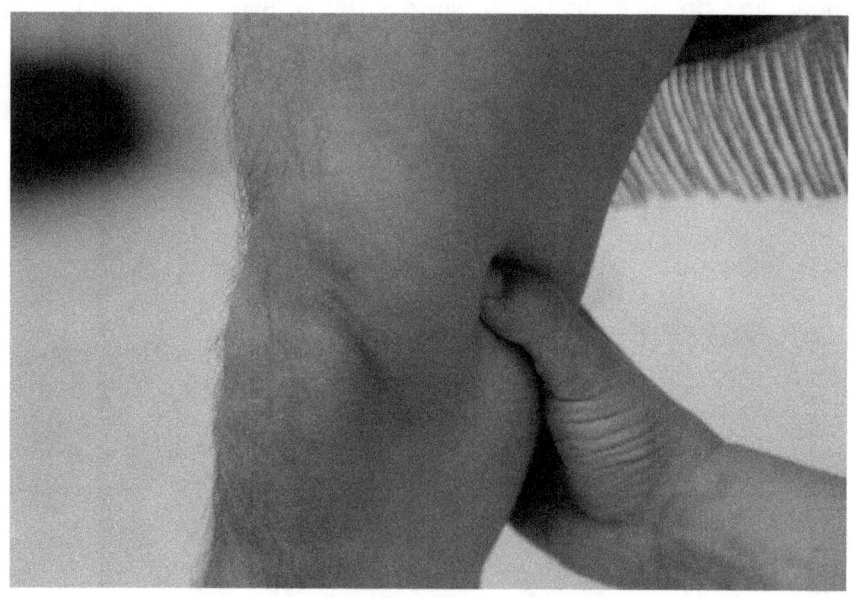

110

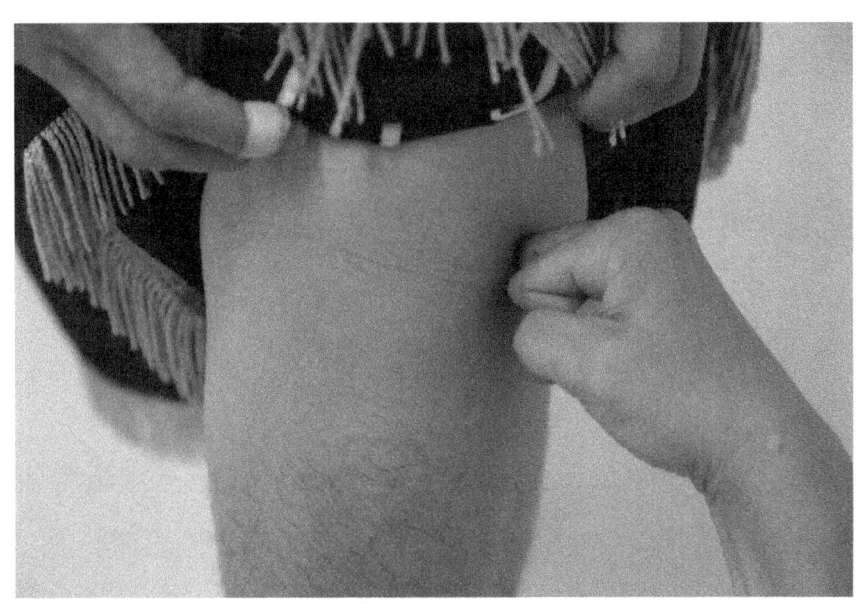

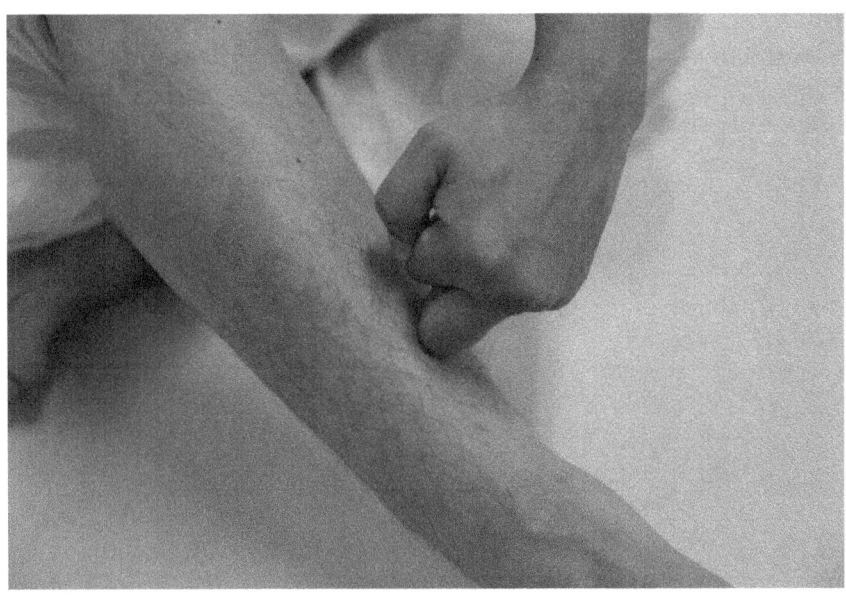

111

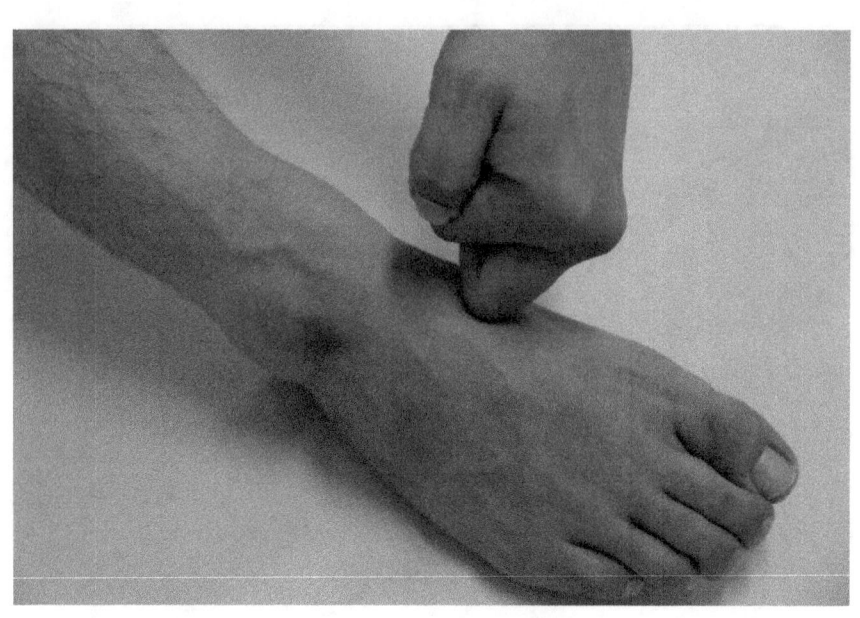

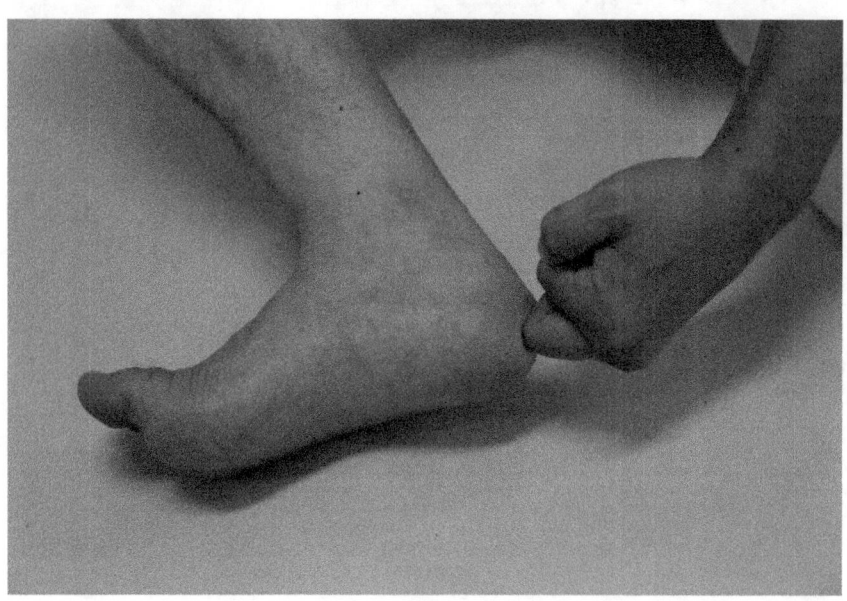

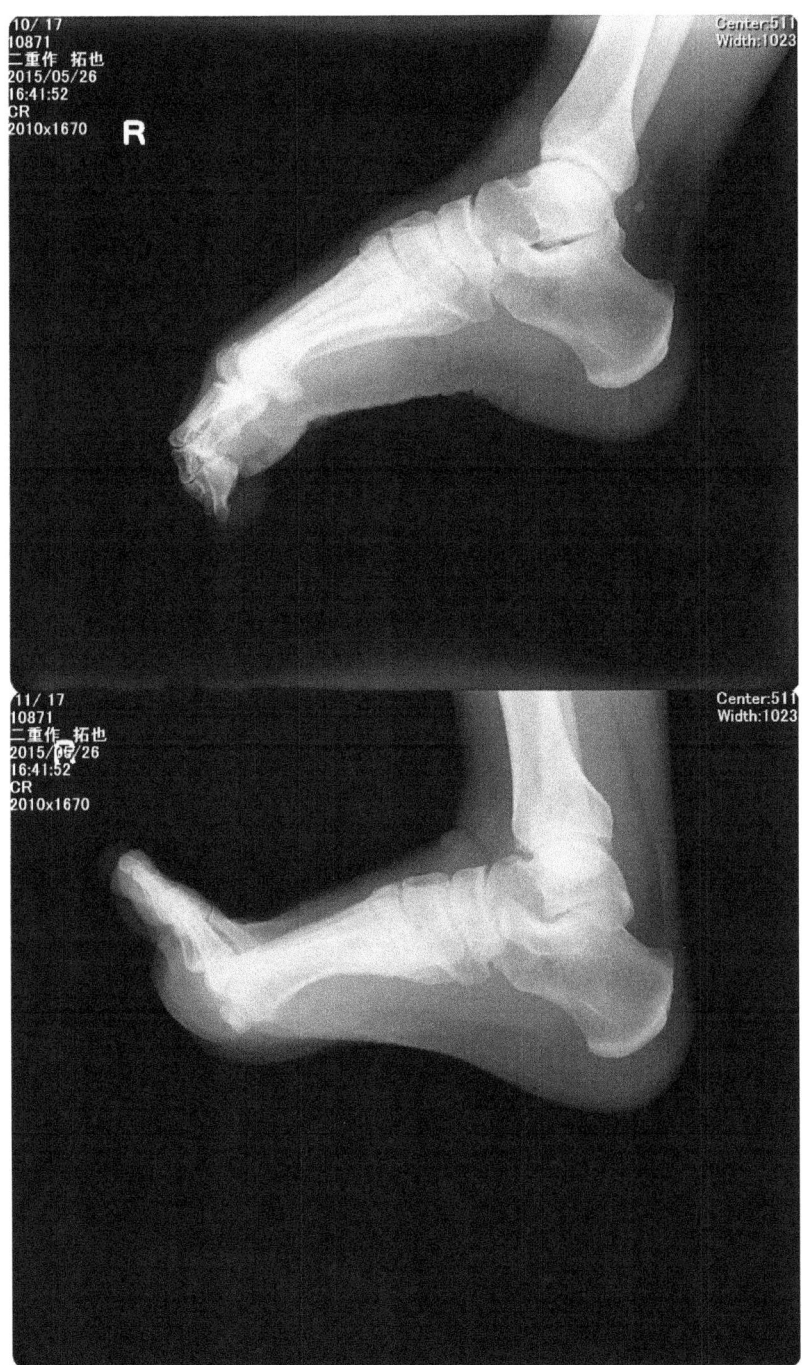

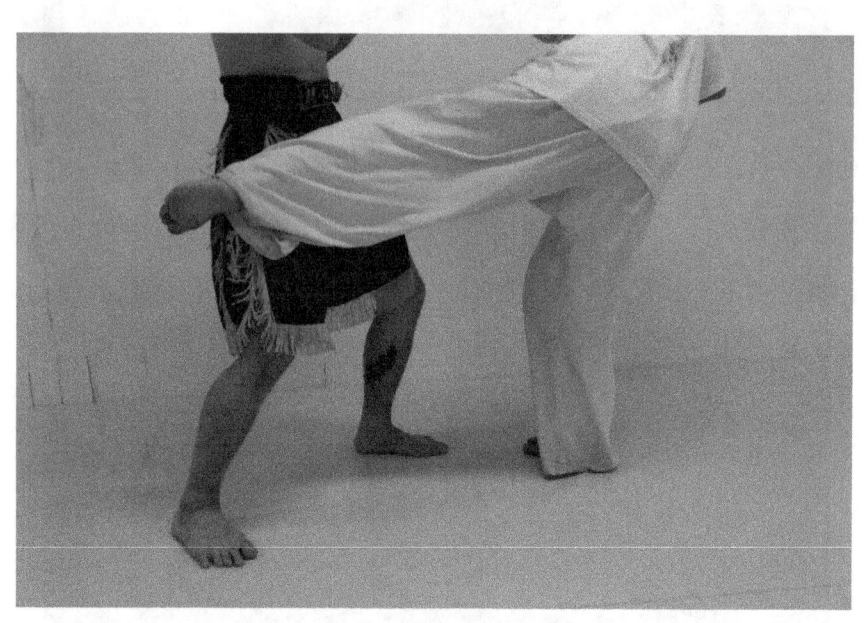

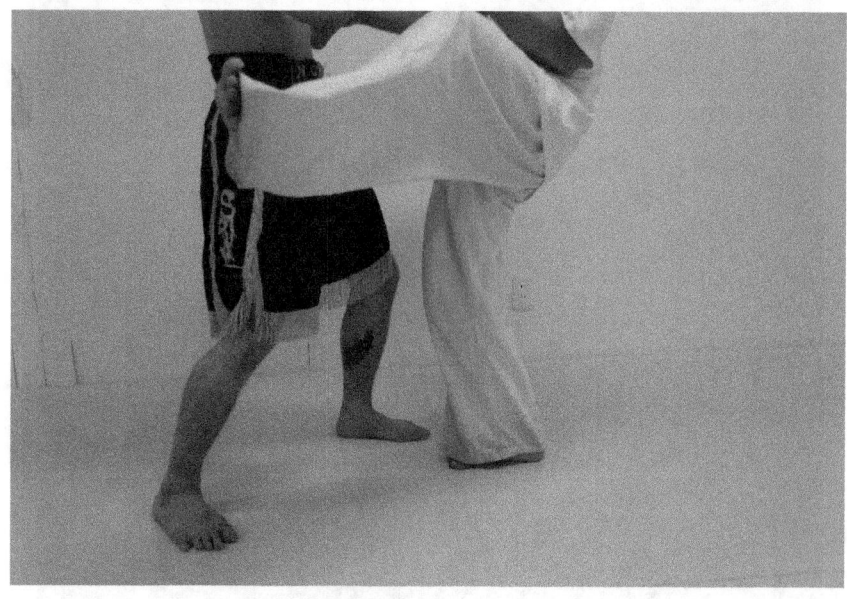

3-7 【Practice through humans】

When you feel a sense of matching points with gedan-geri and low kicks, we will adjust the weak points and strong points in each position to punch, kick, tackle and so on. It doesn't make a fancy sound like "bang", but let's find each other 's feeling like light knock, heavy knock and hard point sticking on the point. When your opponent gives the strike, carefully observe which foot of the opponent is being loaded. For example, an opponent of Orthodox strikes a right straight. At that time, the moment when loading the forefoot (left foot) is a great opportunity to kick the forefoot. Because the opponent's lower limb is fixed to the ground, when the kick is hit, the shock becomes harder to escape and it is easier to damage even the same kick.

In addition, when the opponent's middle kick or the high kick is coming, the opponent's leg also becomes a good target of low kicks. At the moment of defending the kick, the opponent's axis foot tends to point to the right, left side from our side, so it will be easier for our left leg low kick from outside to grasp the point where slightly above the patella, the part where the femur is right under the skin (weak point). Weak points that are difficult to attack on scenes that are in mutual standing will appear in a state that is easy to attack in some skill and movement. If you can accumulate the practice to capture that moment, it will be more likely to lead to KO.

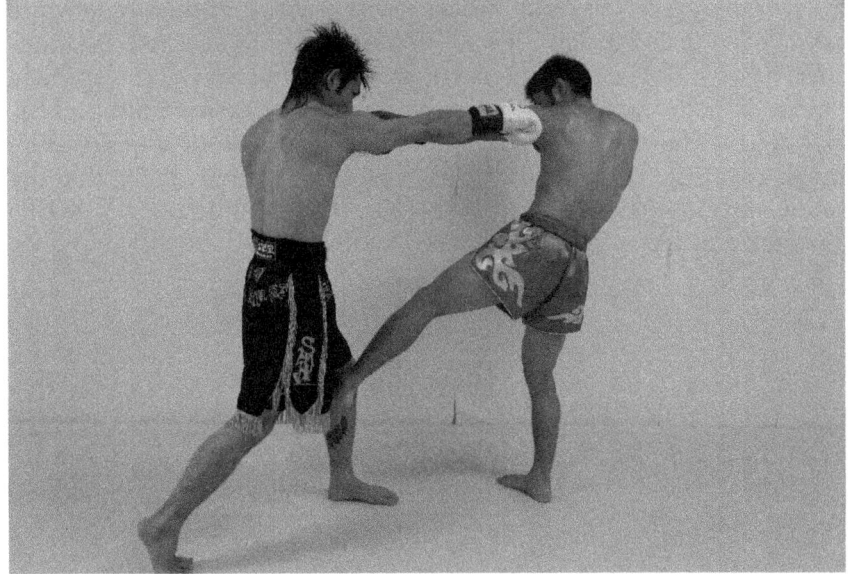

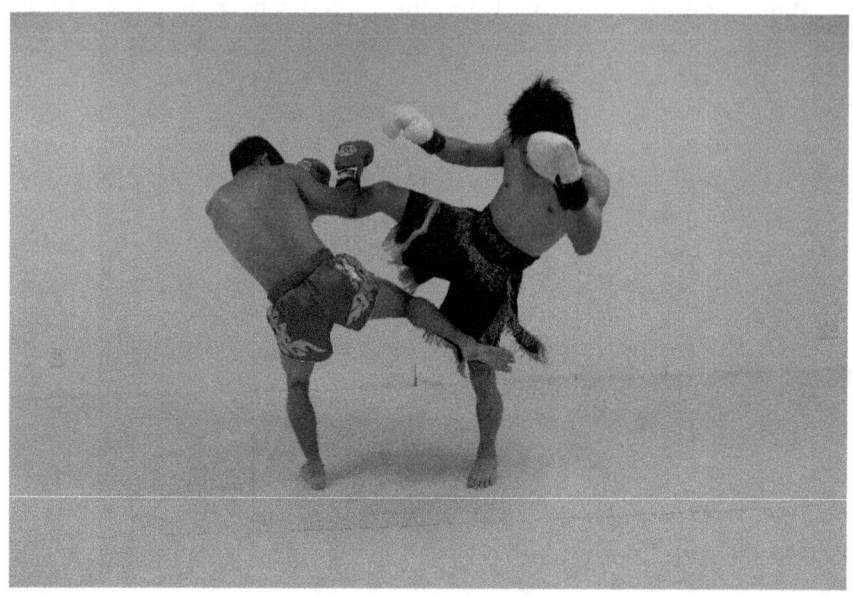

Andy Hug, famous as a specialist of "axe kick". He was a legendary fighter who has been respected by overwhelmingly basic physical strength, precise technology, and challenging spirit, from practitioners all over the world. It is said that his KOs were actually by a lot of low kicks. Of course, there are also matches that KO by hitting the axe kick straight, but using the intense "axe kick", the opponent is scooped down, and at the timing of his loading on the hind leg, then honking down the opponents with the lower kick which follows. It was a feature of Andy that he could continuously carry out two skills with destructive power like axe kick and lower kick which are able to KO.

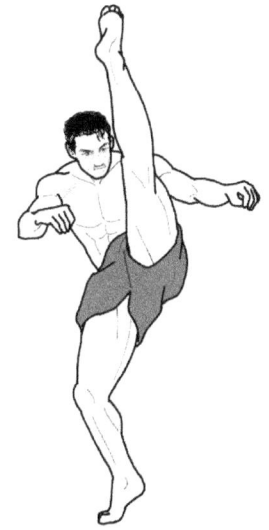

Not only in the low kick, but in strikes, tackles and submissions, there are many people are conscious of "How (how to do)", but "When (which moment to do)" is also very important as a factor. Even if you brush up your skills carefully, it is wasting if you strike when your opponent stands firmly. Have your partner to attack you, and at that moment, where is the point where the lower kick is effective? Which is the load? Which moment is it advantageous to capture? Where is the psychological whitespace or unresponsive time? It is difficult to know by sandbag or mitt practice, and it is hard to be conscious on sparring, so "accumulation of understanding and memory through the human beings" will increase the probability of KO.

3-8 【Invisible things come to be able to see】

It is Westerners who established anatomy. "What about the human body in any way?" People who are interested in it, have interests and doubts have elucidated the details of the inside of the human body and have named on the things no one has named before and systematize them. A thing could be spread only after being named. If it is systematized as academics, everyone can learn correctly. Western medicine that keeps on doing it many years ago and continuing to quantify, visualize, and objectively make them as far as possible today is a tremendous accumulation of collective intelligence. Of course Western medicine and science are not almighty. There are many things that have not been elucidated yet. Rather more things that have not been elucidated. Western medicine and science have the attitude of "trying to elucidate" against what has not yet been elucidated. It is currently moving in a progressive way, including the attitude of trying to construct the methodologies for elucidation. What is going on outside the earth? In response to the question: people invent the method like satellites and rockets, to truly fly out of the earth. It is easy to deny Western medicine and science in words, but they also certainly receive the benefits of medical science and science.

When participants listen to CT images and bone X-ray at study group and seminar of Society of Fighting Medicine, there will be experiences that their movements changes obviously after that. Because after knowing what the contents are like in the CT image, the participants who were randomly kicking the low kicks and gedan-geri become "able to image the running of the femur by seeing the partner's lower limbs". I will shift to a tight language called "kick at one on the medial collateral ligament and the right shinbone" from the ambiguous language "kicking this part like this". And then doing it will actually increase damage to the partner. As the area becomes smaller, the shock given becomes larger, it is a matter of course to study in physics, but in order to realize it, not only do it blindly but know the language → understand the contents → The process of executing it in a language in which contents are aggregated is really effective. Is it possible to increase the reproducibility by storing the movement of low kick in the brain from both the body and the language, both sides.

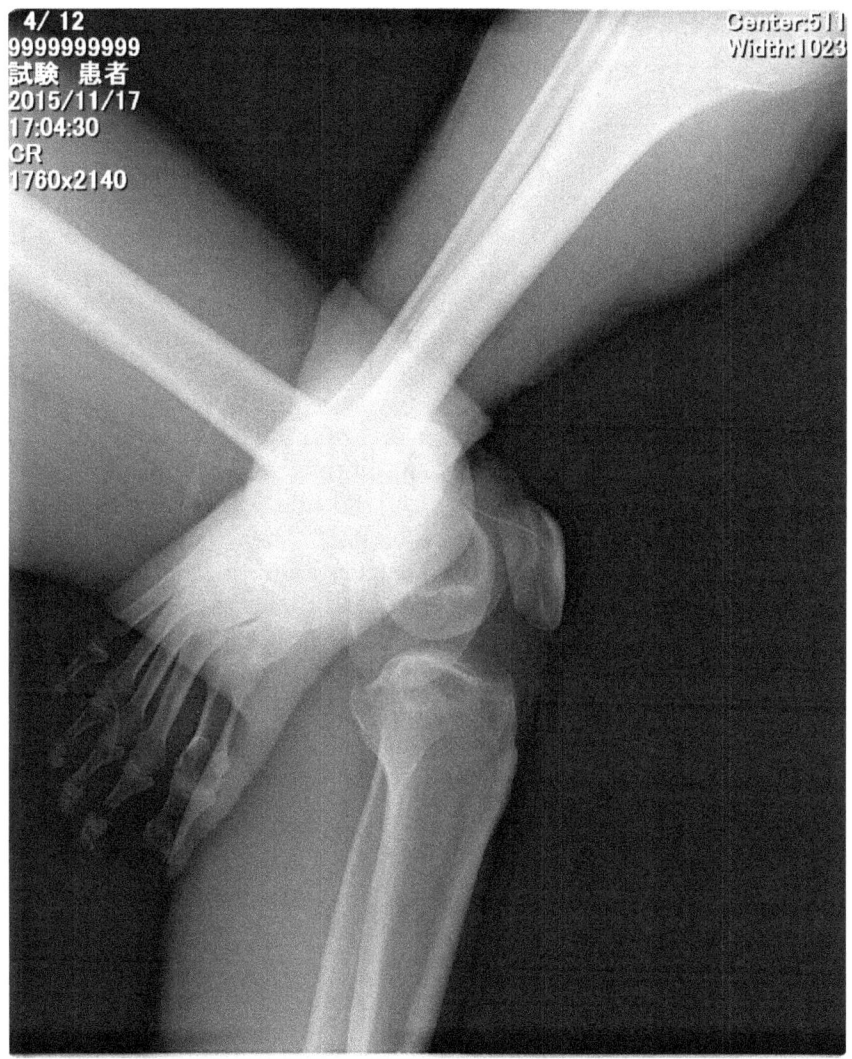

(X-ray :low kick with partner)

In my country, there is still a strong tendency to place emphasis on the succession of traditional performing arts, silently to inherit what we have learned from the teacher and seniors, but overseas fighters and leaders always have the questions "Why?" It seems that they have a strong interest in the Fighting Medicine approach. They stare at the CT images and ask me more and more questions. I want to know, passion to want to be strong, no, even in obsession, I feel that overseas forces surpass us Japanese. In Western medicine and science, both blood pressure and blood glucose level have been quantified. As a result, we can understand the state with numbers, and we can take appropriate measures and evaluations instantaneously. "When blood pressure has returned to the normal range if you regularly exercise after being careful of your diet", what will you obtain from it? That's "Health" and "Confidence". If you do it properly, you can see the result. "somehow good feeling" could be proven.Also in the low kick, "If at this timing, this part is damaged if you hit this part of the shin against the region of the greater trochanter" to improve it while repeating trial and error, when it did not go well You can review each element individually. People who have done with so-called sense alone are hard to notice the difference in something, so there are many cases that cannot quite get out of slumps, but those who have tried to improve by trial and error, they have the check points in the brain and the body, so the corrections will be easier. In addition, based on the structure and principle of human beings, the direction to develop original skills and tactics could be also born. Science and medicine make it easy to see invisible things, make it easier to imagine the invisible part beyond the boundary line, and are strong friends that will promote the reproducibility of know-how.

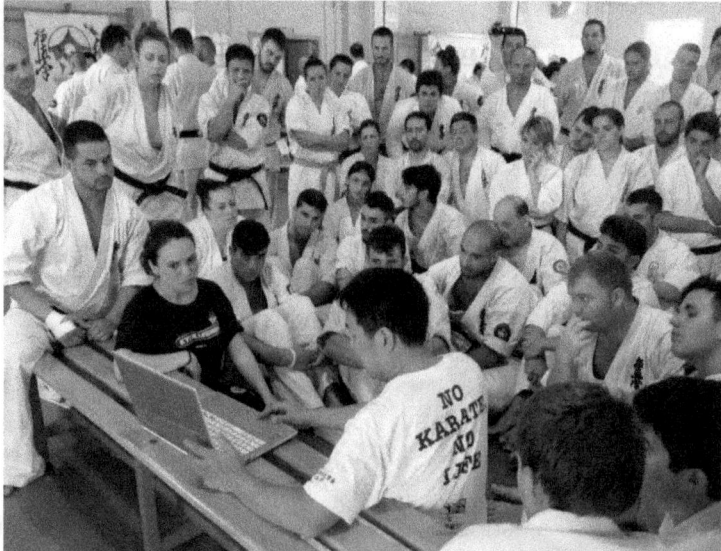

(Kyokushin WKB summner camp in Spain)

4:What Is KO?
-KO sense-

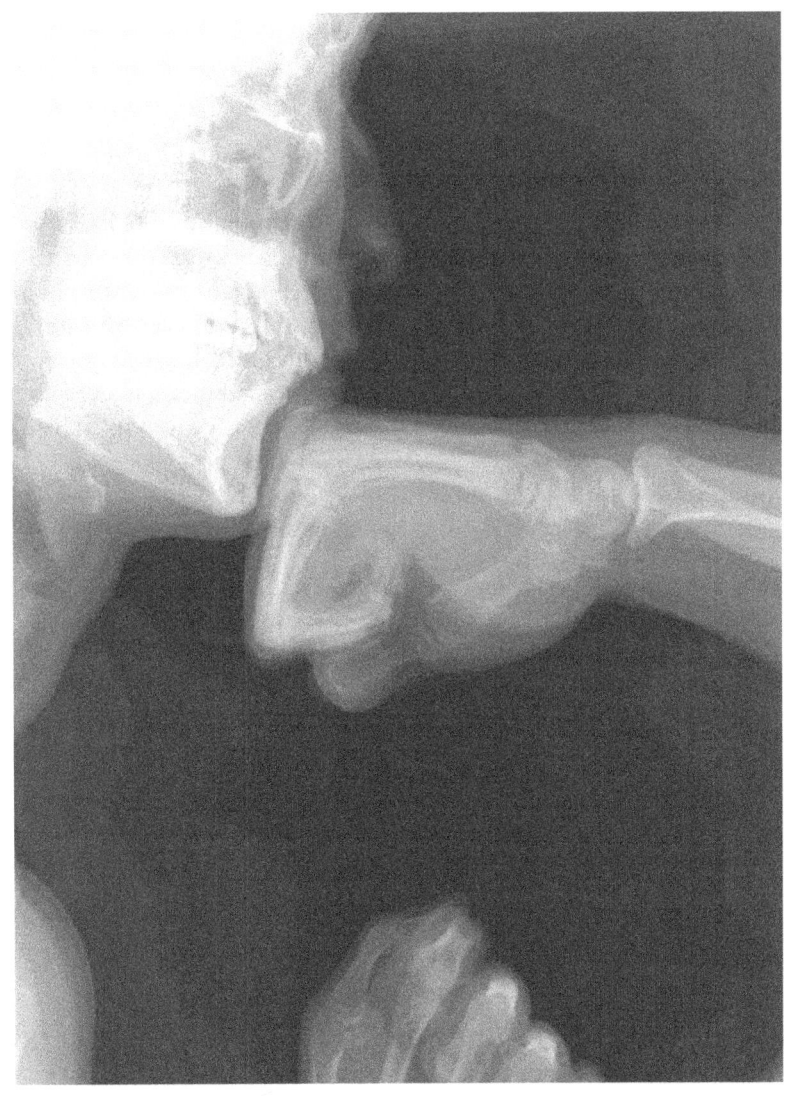

4-1 【What is the biggest reason why you cannot knockdown the opponent? 】

"How do I get the skills to KO?"

It was a long-standing question as a practitioner. Regardless of the place in a match, I can not afford to KO important friends and juniors of the same dojo. If your brain already has a feeling and memory of KO in the game, even if you have a mitt or bag in front of you, you can practice while linking with the memory when you KO a human, but if the memory of KO is not accumulated in your brain, it is hard to make the image of KO itself. Besides that, in my case, there was a tendency to be pulled by objects in front of my eyes. I punch and kick the mitt in front of me, it becomes the kicks to the object instead of the human body. While looking for the difference between the fighter whom can knockdown and the fighter who cannot, the fighter I noticed the fighters whom cannot knockdown, there are not a few practitioners who accumulated the erroneous memory that "Even if my blow is hit, the opponent will not be knocked down". "Even if you win by judgment it is difficult, even if you win, so waza-ari and ippon are the dreams in a dream",

placing KO too high priority on the top, so there are many people do not pursue KO or give up KO from the beginning.

It is completely different if "It's to practice a high kick by thinking it can knockdown" and "It's to practice a high kick while doubting, that it wouldn't knockdown anyway." I like the person and looking directly at the his/her eyes and hating the person and staring his/her eyes are not the same even that's the same gesture to look at his/her eyes but different meanings aren't they? In creating a skill, the image pops up in the brain reflects the movement of the body as it is. How can I train the feeling of knockdown? After the pursuit of this theme then and finally completed, that is the KO training bag.

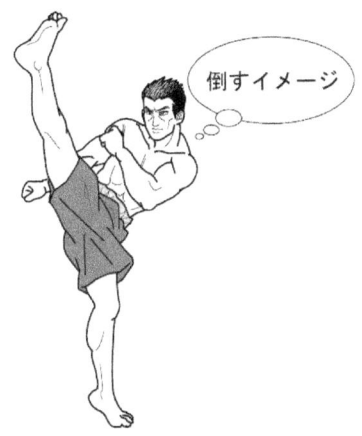

(KO image)

4-2 【Reduce exercise becoming weaken】

A normal sandbag has a considerable weight, it does not move very much, even if you punch or kick, its shape does not change either. For example, when practicing a combination that knocks down with a high kick after kicking a knee kick from a one-two punch, a high kick does not hit the sandbag unless you get back to the initiating distance once, before hitting the high kick. If you practice it many times, that will settle into your brain and become a habit, while you do not realize "movement that goes back all the way though the knee kick hit". At the game, the opponent comes forward at the moment you are going back by yourself, and you cannot kick a high kick and gets caught by the opponent. You are practicing that habit.

For the KO by the head attack, we want to shake the brain at the maximum speed at the moment that the strike hits, but when it hits late, it will be difficult for a concussion to happen. If it is a heavy-duty bag, its feedback certainly is big, but as soon as it meets the surface, the speed approaches zero. If you repeat this, there is a possibility that even in the actual match, you cannot get out of the habit of stopping the technique and you might be missing out the KO opportunity. The biggest problem of these weakening exercises is that the principal who is doing it does not notice the case.

4-3 【Bringing in the medical essence】

We are bringing in the anatomical figures into the KO training bag. The width of the KO bag adopts almost the same value as the width of the base point of the Japanese chin and the position just in the middle of the tip, also about the length, this is also from the top of a general Japanese head to the bottom of the neck, it's made about twice as long. When a strike hits, it is a design that bends like "L" shape, so you can evaluate the completeness of the technique visually and objectively. If the bag turns into a "L" shape, the strike is going through sharply, and if the shape of the sandbag remains unchanged as it is, it means that the speed and impact of the strike could be further extended. Also, as we mentioned above, when we kick your opponent in a match, we often experience unexpectedly little resistance on your hand or leg. In this bag, the reaction is much smaller than the heavy bag, so you get a feeling close to the blow when you shake your opponent's brain.

In the world of medicine, there is a training to have a patient who cannot walk wear a walking device like a robot, and walk with help of the external force, to regain the "sense of walking" in the nervous system. Apart from you can or you can't, by setting a possible state, inputting "sense of being capable" in the brain and fix it. KO Bag certainly is for people who can KO, but also the aim is to get the feeling of knock down, especially for those who wish to make a KO come true. If you can punch or kick to deform it into "L" shape, at least the speed at the moment you hit is not zero, so I think that it will lead to increase the ratio of the possibility to KO. "The feeling of being able to walk, for a person who cannot walk" "The feeling of being able to knockdown for a person who can't knockdown the opponent" The aim is to transform the feeling of the brain and nurture confidence to be able to do it.

In the case of exercises aiming to KO with a body blow, wrap a soft blanket or mat around the circumference, give a difference in hardness, and strike its deep part. With gedan-geri and low kick, attach a mark of a point with a taping etc., and train a blow that sandwiches a pain spot between a point and a point. With the

124

kicking of the surface, the bag moves greatly, but because the bag deforms with the point kick, it is easy to evaluate with visuals.

In the competition where close skill level fighters are fighting, it is rare that a fighter whom doesn't move knocks down a fighter who moves. It is meaningful for a fighter who can move doesn't move, but if that was not able to move, it is quite far from being able to KO. Also, no matter how much you can do your technics, without the supporting power or stamina, it will not be conveyed to your opponent as power.

KO bag, and his younger brother, KO Bag Extra, gained unprecedented mobility by connecting it to a tube. Since there are parts that can be connected to the underside of the KO Bag Extra, kick mitts and tubes can be connected there, so depending on the ingenuity, it becomes a troublesome "opponent" that is hard to control. Like a rugby ball, it moves unexpectedly, so it will be "can't control how I want" load. This is close to the feeling of the match. Also, normal sandbag hangs vertically in the direction of gravity, but KO Bag Extra can set at random such as diagonal and horizontal. We looked to respond to "evolving technology" that had not existed several decades, such as axe kick, Brazilian high kick, inner kick, wheel kick, heel kick.

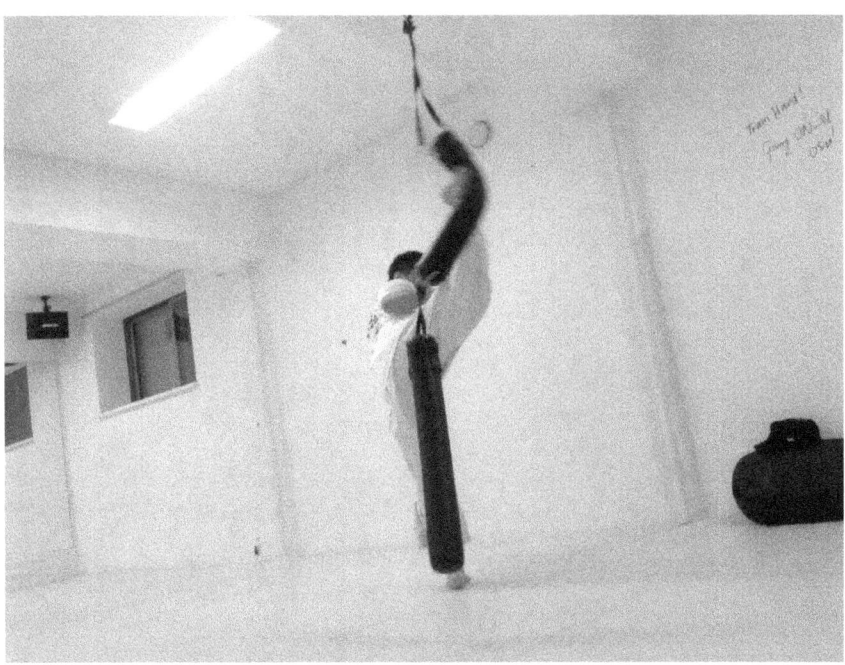

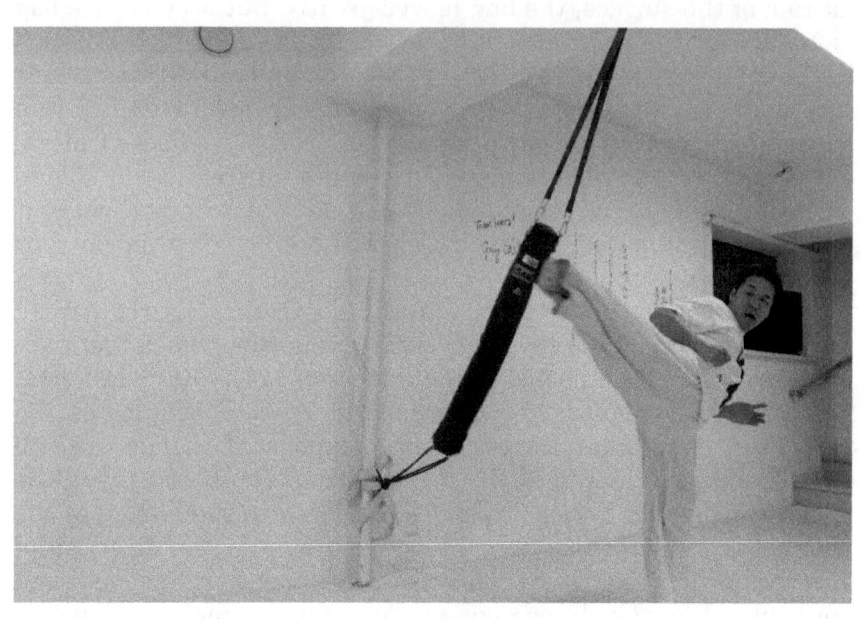

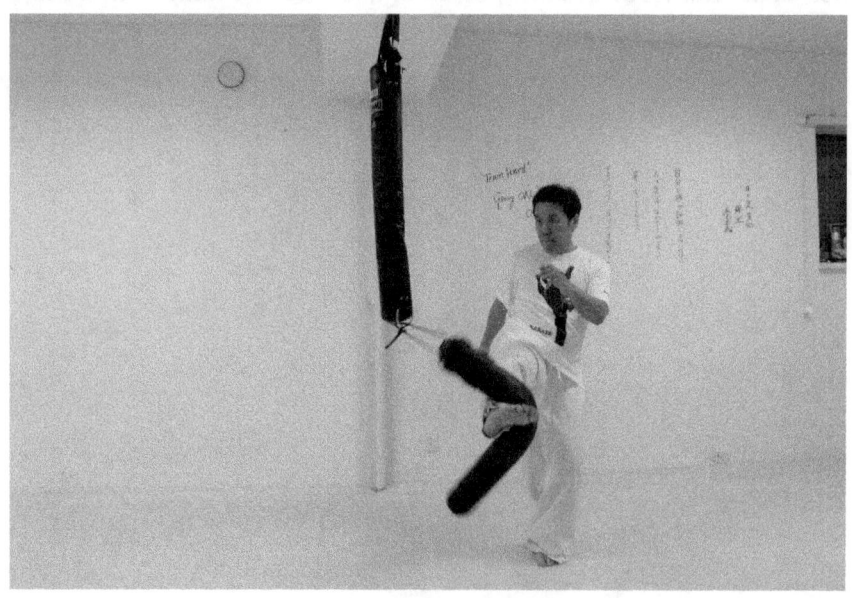

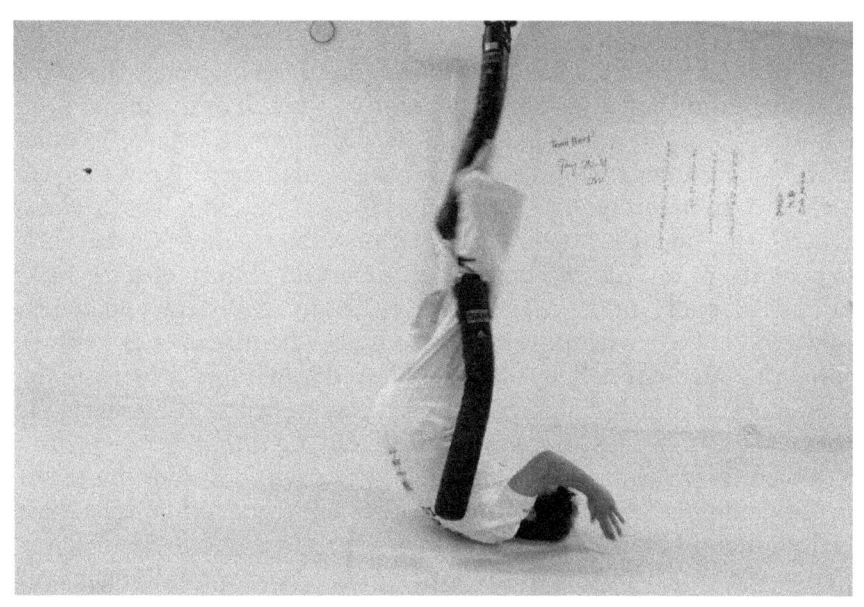

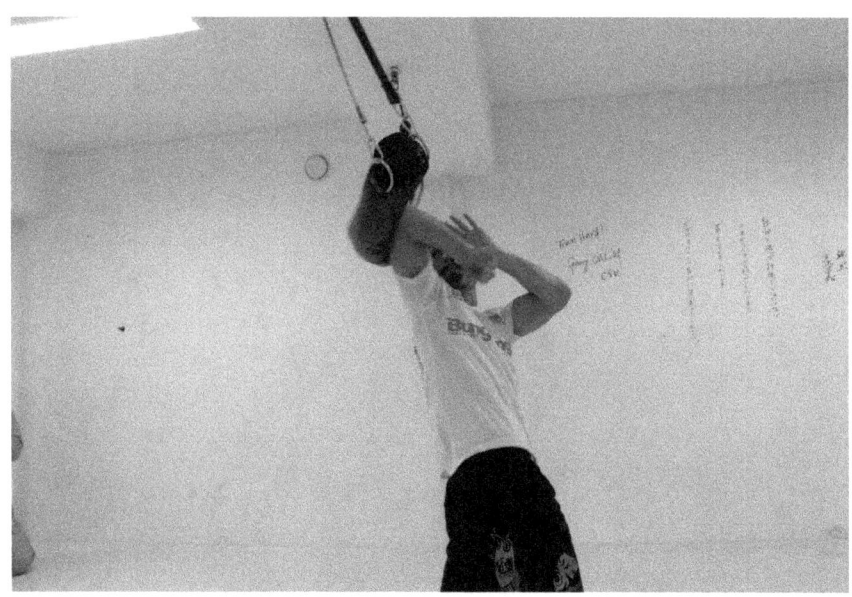

4-4 【One & only style】

Considering what load is necessary to become strong, the work of embodying that idea is a very creative work. For example, even with the same high kick, the high kick of the long legged fighter's high kick against the opponent and the short legged fighter's high kick are completely different. In the case of long leg fighters, control the opponent at a long distance, the moment when the opponent enters his own control of air is the chance of high kick, in the case of short legged fighters, jump into the opponent's control of the air with punch or so to make the distance as close as zero, the moment when the opponent doesn't like it and make some distance, is the chance of high kick. In order to increase the chance of a high kick in a limited time during a match, the former is a technic which does not let the opponent gets inside, the latter is the technic of getting inside the opponent's guard and inner low kick and body blows, or tackle to position down the head which is the target of hitting, become important. Even just talking about high kick, there are variations of choice depending on the conditions such as the physical characteristics of yourself, the position of your physique in the competition, the relationship with the opponent.

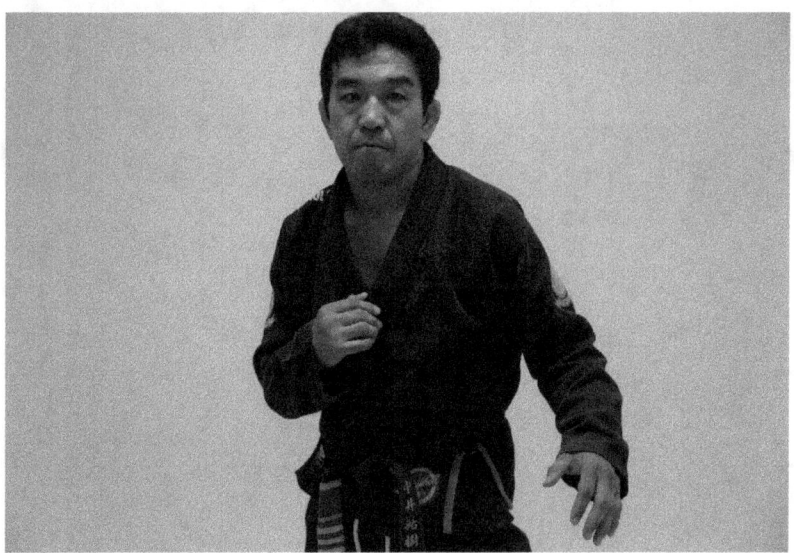

(Mr.Yuuki Nakai)

A legendary fighter, Yuuki Nakai (PARAESTRA Tokyo), who

has fought in real earnest with that Rickson Gracie and has pioneered mixed martial arts and jiu-jitsu, said, "The style of fighting sports, everyone is original. There is no other same style" as he expresses. Indeed, many top players are creating a way to make themselves stronger by themselves. The technique itself is not originally there, but someone creates and then generalized body control, so the technics will continue to diversify more and more even from now on. If a skill that no one has seen is completed, it is a threat to the opponent. Creating is important to the partner to generate a state that "I don't know what he/she is doing on me". It is not an unusual style that simply got strange, but one and only creative style that swallowed several royal roads will further evolve fighting sports and martial arts.

4-5 【Fixing memory of being able to do】

I talked about the anatomy section of KO of gedan-geri and low kick, but if you realize the KO in the match, there is something you certainly want you to carry out. That is to make language of KO situation as much as possible. How long since the start of the match, where in the ring, how you were moving, how the opponent was moving, what voice you were hiring, what scene was getting in your sight, what you were feeling, what kind of process the strike popped out, what kind of feeling you had at the moment you knockdown the opponent, what you though at that moment, etc. Mark down the memory of KO with literal words, reconstruct in conversational words, to your juniors or your trustable partners, with gestures, to reproduce the scene in interpersonal. In a won match, information input is done. Since the channel is open, the loop of sensory input → processing information → output via motor nerve → sensory input, is well behaved. In a lost match we are fed up, fall into the narrowing of the field of vision, almost no voice of the second is heard. In order to achieve high randomness KO or highly repeatable KO, it is effective to fix the feeling and situation when KO was made, into the brain. Through conversion to output and language. Then you will find out that KO's opportunity has come when you are in a similar situation. Even a test question of mathematics to be seen for the first time is similar to a process which makes it easier to get to the right answer when you see closely and finds that similar problems and structures are common issues that have been done in the past. It is also important to verbalize not only KO but also the experience of winding patterns and pinch over. In the era of overinformation, there are lots of tips outside of you, but the answer is in yourself. If you use letters and pictures to right down the notes about what that is about, you can create your own reinforcement textbook. If you do not accumulate "memory of not being able to" but "memory of being able to" carefully and certainly like bricks, you will surely get closer to KO.

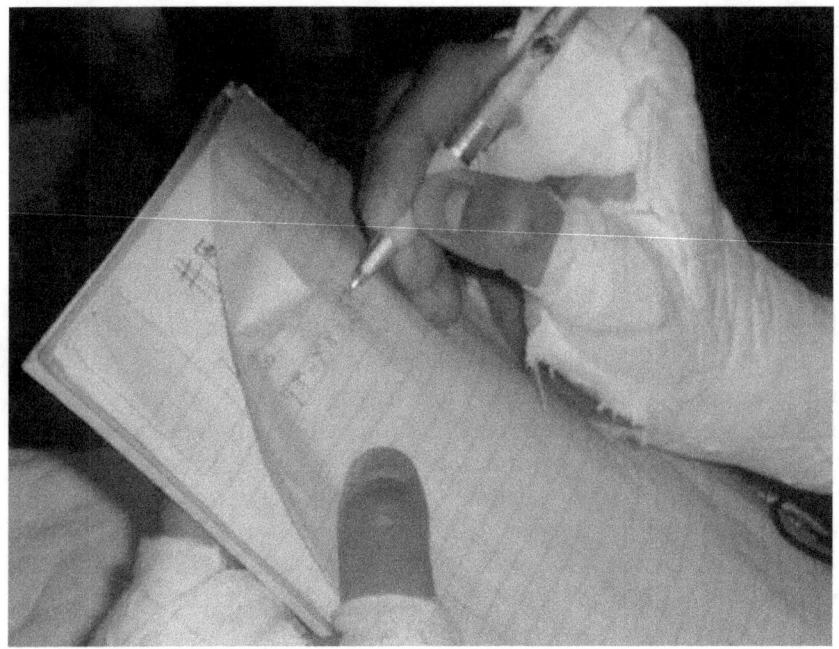

--- End---

Recommendation

UFC fighter, Kiichi Kunimoto

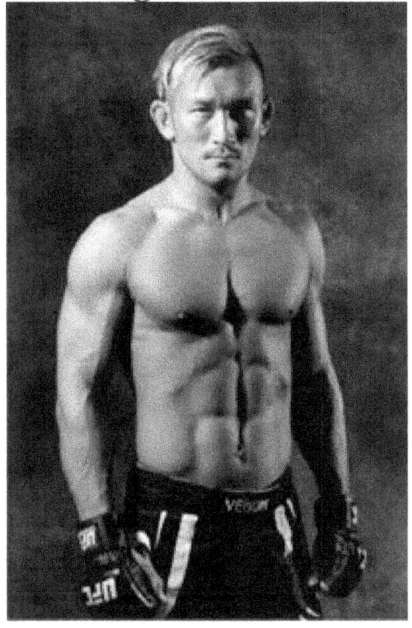

The time I first met Dr. Futaesaku was not much later than I became a professional fighter. I placed my base in Tokyo, and learnt a lot of how to use the body and brain, as well as techniques and the image trainings. Every single time I had an inspiration and could meet a new myself. We made our goals. Me as "Fighting in the best qualified arena called UFC", Dr.F as "Spread the Fighting Medicine to the world wide" Had been cooperating each other and working hard on each side throughly. and with a luck, my debut came true in January 2014. 3 wins straight. I have since been feeling my improvement. If you have a will of wanting to be stronger even a tiny bit more than now, I strongly, fully recommend this

100 men fights achiever, Karate legend Kancho Ademir Da Costa

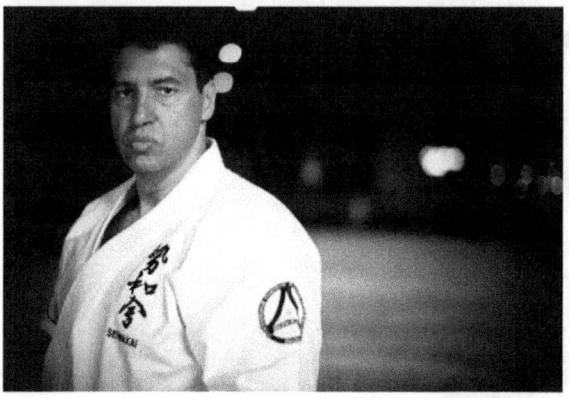

I congratulate Dr. F for his incredible work for the health of the practitioners of the martial arts. His scientific research about the best way to prevent injuries in hard training - which the athletes are submitted - and the correct way to practice some techniques, will help both professional fighters as the beginners, to have health and quality of live. I suffered many injuries caused by the hard trainings without any scientific orientation. Now, with the research of Dr.F, the new generation of practitioners of martial arts will have a correct orientation to practice the martial arts with a healthy way. My sincere thanks for this as important work for the martial art and budo. Osu!

Kyokushin WKB CEO, Kancho Pedro Roiz

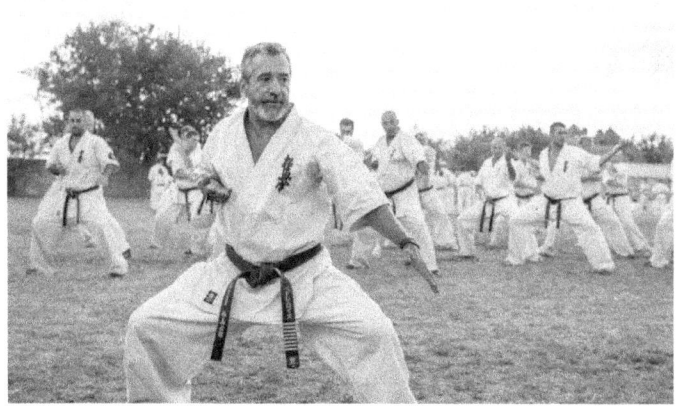

This book has been well received within the martial arts community and I especially cannot recommend this amazingly well researched and well written book enough. Fightology is possibly the best scientifically written martial arts book to be published. Reading this book will open new doors to the execution of techniques and will give a better understanding of our Martial Arts. Through its pages we will get a better work foundation to achieve greater results in our athletes and, furthermore, a better understanding of how the internal energy works. This exquisite book is the result of years of exhaustive work, carried out by the preparation and the scientific rigor of a doctor, combined with the first-hand experiences of a martial artist. Dr.F is a lover of these arts, and his insatiable hunger for researching allowed him to contact some of the most reputed teachers, with whom he has worked extensively in the study of body motion. He is not just a scientist with sufficient basic knowledge of anatomy, physiology... to carry out this deepening task. He is also "one of us", able to address this study from our perspective, from the knowledge of a martial artist. And this is what makes the analysis much more adjusted to our demand. From these lines and from the great affection I have for him, I would like to express my appreciation and admiration for this great work, wishing Dr.F all the success he deserves, and hoping that he always keeps that clean gesture on his face.

MMA legend &
Arm wrestling World Champ
Gary Goodridge

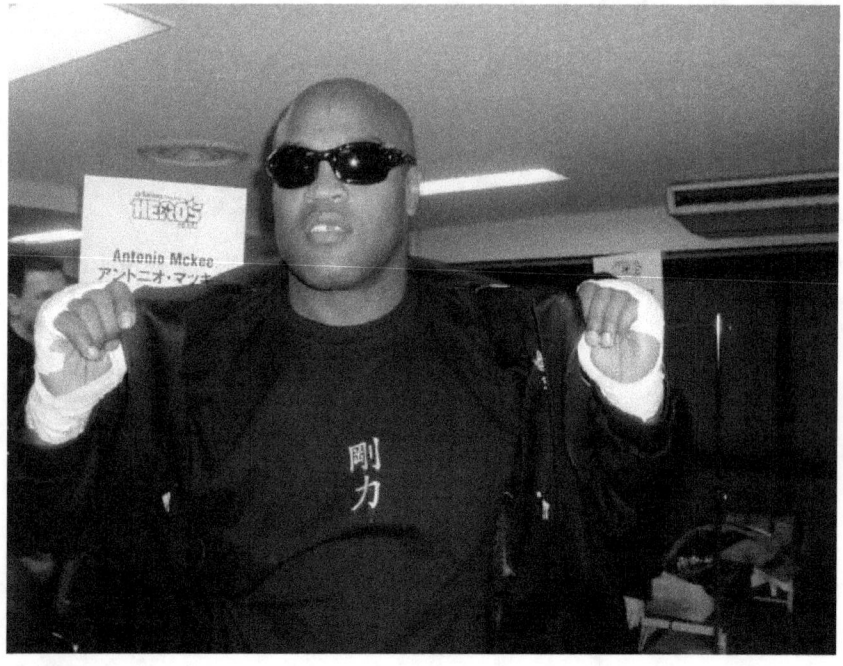

Dr.F was my team doctor as I was a professional fighter for a few years. Worked my corner on several different occasions. I am sure he will be more then competent to do any job as helping out in MMA or any fighting organizations.

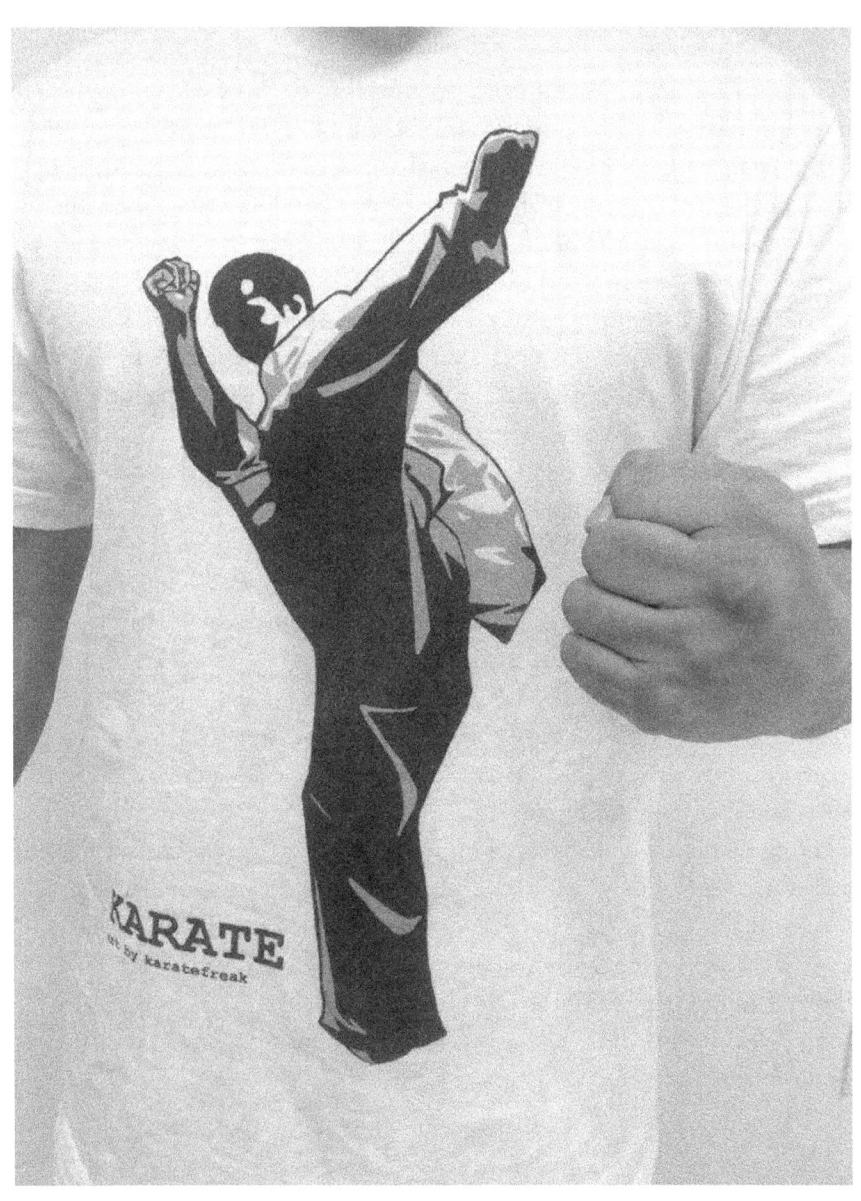

Takuya Futaesaku (a.k.a "Dr.F")

is a Sports Medicine Doctor from Japan famous for his work in supporting many professional fighting sports athletes from Karate, Muay Thai / Kickboxing, and MMA. Dr.F developed a strong interest in the martial arts since he was a child. He initially began training in full-contact Karate and became a Karate instructor during his high school years. While studying at Kochi Medical School (Kochi University), his enthusiasm for fighting sports led him to apply his medical knowledge (such as anatomy, kinetics, kinesiology, etc.), using the term - "Fightology" to encompass his medical research on Fighting sports. His medical science approach in fighting sports is a very new and exciting concept, with his work attracting attention from martial arts enthusiasts around the world. His "Fightology" seminars, which have been held in Australia, Europe, Chile, Costa Rica, and Hong Kong, have been very popular and in turn recognizing Dr. F as a true innovator in fighting sports. Aside from his "Fightology" seminars, Dr.F is also a famous contributor for various Japanese sport magazines such as Ironman magazine, Full Contact Karate, Coaching Clinic and more recently Fight and Life magazine. He is also the author of "Fighting Sports for Juniors", "Medical Science Of Fighting Sports" "Self improving Training learning from Top Fighters" and the DVD producer of "The Anatomy of Knockout Vol1&2", and "The Kinematics of Fighting Sports Vol.1 to 7" - all of his works are ranked 5 stars on Amazon Japan. Today, Dr.F continues to develop "Fightology" with medical knowledge, research, and passion. He is looking forward to raising the level for combat sports enthusiasts all around the world. He is also recognized as music tour doctor, Supporting Prince family, George Clinton &P-funk, Tower Of Power, Candy Dulfer, John Blackwell and more top artists. His book about Prince, Words Of Prince" is also best seller in Japan.

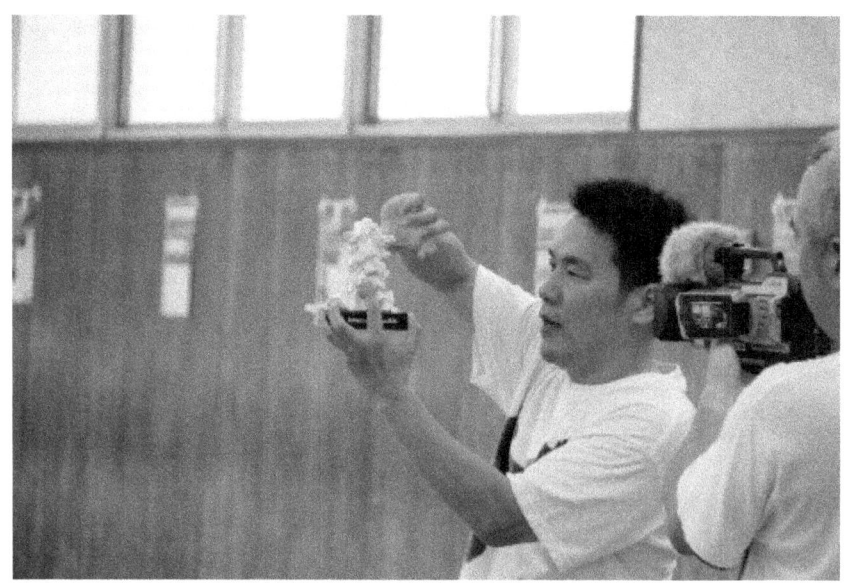

<Contact & Booking>

No Karate No Life official page
https://www.facebook.com/nokaratenolife

Facebook
https://www.facebook.com/takuya.futaesaku

Instagram
https://www.instagram.com/takuyafutaesaku/

ありがとうございました。
Thank you very much

押忍
Dr. F

September 2017

www.ingramcontent.com/pod-product-compliance
Lightning Source LLC
Chambersburg PA
CBHW051537170526
45165CB00002B/768